Dr. Barbara O'Neill's Ancient Book of Revived Herbal Remedies

4 Books in 1

A Better You Everyday Publications
Email: info@abetteryoueveryday.com

Disclaimer

The information provided in this book is for educational and informational purposes only and is not affiliated with, authorized, endorsed by, or in any way officially connected with Barbara O'Neill or her affiliates or subsidiaries. The use of Barbara O'Neill's name in this book is for explanatory, educational, and reference purposes only, to discuss and provide insight into the theories and practices she has publicized through her teachings and public appearances. The views and interpretations presented in this book solely reflect those of the author and have not been reviewed or approved by Barbara O'Neill or her representatives.

The content within this book is not intended as medical advice and should not be taken as such. The author, Margaret Willowbrook, is not a medical professional. This book should not replace consultation with a qualified healthcare professional. It is essential that before beginning any new health practice, you consult with your physician, especially if you have any pre-existing health conditions.

While every effort has been made to verify the information provided in this book, the field of natural health is dynamic, and as such, the content may not reflect the most recent research or medical consensus. The author and publisher assume no responsibility for errors, omissions, or contrary interpretations of the subject matter herein.

Readers are encouraged to confirm the information contained within this publication through independent research and professional advice. Any perceived slights of specific people or organizations are unintentional. By reading this book, you agree that the author and publisher are not responsible for the success or failure of your health decisions related to any information presented.

A Better You
Everyday Publications

info@abetteryoueveryday.com

www.abetteryoueveryday.com

Dr. Barbara O'Neill's Ancient Book of Revived Herbal Remedies 4 Books in 1

600+ Holistic Cures, Teas, Balms, Essential Oils, and Natural Antibiotics for Complete Modern Healing Inspired by Her Teachings

By

Margaret Willowbrook

USA 2024

Table of Contents

Introduction

The Life, Teachings, and Philosophy of Dr. Barbara O'Neill

Dr. Barbara O'Neill, an Australian wellness advocate and self-described naturopath, has spent years promoting a philosophy centered on the body's ability to heal itself. Her approach is rooted in the idea that natural remedies, lifestyle changes, and environmental factors like fresh air, sunlight, and water play essential roles in achieving wellness. O'Neill's teachings stress that health can be maintained, and ailments alleviated by aligning oneself with nature's rhythms. Her methods appeal to those seeking alternatives to conventional medicine, encouraging individuals to take control of their health through natural interventions and lifestyle adjustments.

O'Neill's teachings have continued to reach audiences worldwide, especially through social media platforms where her philosophy of self-healing and empowerment through natural means has found significant resonance. Her ideas draw from a broad spectrum of alternative healing practices, advocating for holistic health as a counter to the perceived shortcomings of conventional medical treatments. Dr. O'Neill emphasizes that nature provides us with an accessible pharmacy, and it is her mission to educate others on using these resources to achieve sustainable wellness.

The Journey into Herbal Medicine and Natural Healing

Dr. O'Neill's journey in naturopathy and herbal medicine has been a gradual evolution from conventional understandings of health to holistic approaches. While she began her career grounded in modern health care frameworks, her focus shifted to natural remedies and lifestyle changes as the primary means of maintaining health. Dr. O'Neill's exploration led her to advocate practices from various healing traditions, including some teachings from Traditional Chinese Medicine and Ayurvedic systems. However, her advocacy has been controversial due to her lack of formal qualifications and her promotion of methods that conflict with evidence-based medical advice.

Her philosophy asserts that prevention, self-awareness, and intentional living are key to achieving a state of holistic wellness. However, Dr. O'Neill's promotion of treatments such as bicarbonate of soda for cancer and unpasteurized goat's milk for infants, both of which are scientifically unsupported and potentially harmful, has drawn significant criticism. Despite this, her work persists in alternative health communities that view her teachings as a return to traditional practices in which nature serves as both protector and healer. Dr. O'Neill's followers embrace her message that health can be maintained through natural rhythms, herbs, and lifestyle adjustments, even as critics urge caution when considering these methods.

Core Beliefs in Holistic Wellness

Central to Dr. Barbara O'Neill's approach is the belief that holistic health stems from balance and prevention. Her philosophy advocates for proactive wellness by nurturing physical, emotional, and mental well-being through mindful, natural practices. Rather than focusing solely on symptom relief, Dr. O'Neill encourages an approach that addresses root causes, advocating for lifestyle choices that strengthen immunity, restore vitality, and support overall resilience. This perspective underscores the idea that health is sustained through thoughtful choices, including nutrient-dense foods, herbal remedies, and preventive care routines, all of which align with the body's natural functions.

Dr. Barbara O'Neill's Ancient Book of Revived Herbal Remedies: 4 Books in 1 serves as a comprehensive guide, offering over 600 natural solutions across a broad spectrum of health needs. Divided into four distinct books, this volume provides readers with accessible, proven methods for natural healing. Book 1 focuses on holistic cures and natural antibiotics to help the body's defenses against common infections and imbalances. Book 2 delves into the art of herbal teas and non-alcoholic tinctures to promote vitality and well-being. Book 3 introduces essential oils and balms, exploring their applications in both physical care and emotional support. Finally, Book 4 presents preventive health practices and daily routines, empowering readers with strategies for consistent, long-term wellness.

Within this 4-in-1 guide, each chapter is crafted to be both informative and practical. Readers will find actionable guidance on preparing remedies, understanding dosages, and integrating natural healing practices into everyday life. From immune-boosting tonics and restorative teas to topical balms for pain relief and mental clarity, this book is designed to empower readers with the knowledge and tools needed to build a natural, balanced approach to health. For those seeking to explore a pathway to wellness rooted in nature, this book provides a wealth of resources to support and sustain well-being.

Reconnecting with Nature for Self-Healing

At a time when many feel disconnected from the natural world, Dr. O'Neill's work emphasizes a return to nature-based wellness practices. Her teachings invite readers to reconnect with the earth's rhythms and resources, and offer practical ways to incorporate natural remedies into daily life. With over 600 remedies, including teas, balms, essential oils, and antibiotics, the book provides readers with tangible ways to support health at every stage, from respiratory wellness and digestive support to emotional balance and relaxation.

Each practice encourages readers to embrace natural remedies as reliable tools for personal care.

Ancient Book of Revived Herbal Remedies provides a complete foundation for individuals seeking to care for their physical, mental, and emotional well-being. Each section of the book emphasizes practical, actionable steps that readers can take to address their unique health needs. By the end of the book, readers will have discovered a full range of holistic strategies for cultivating resilience and health. Through easy-to-follow recipes, detailed insights, and accessible language, this guide allows readers to confidently explore self-healing practices that align with natural rhythms and principles.

In addition to serving as a health resource, this book encourages readers to view wellness as an ongoing journey. Dr. O'Neill's philosophy goes beyond remedies to promote a mindset of self-awareness, intentionality, and respect for the body's natural healing abilities. Readers will find this comprehensive guide not only a source of practical information, but also an invitation to cultivate lasting habits of care that can contribute to a lifetime of wellness.

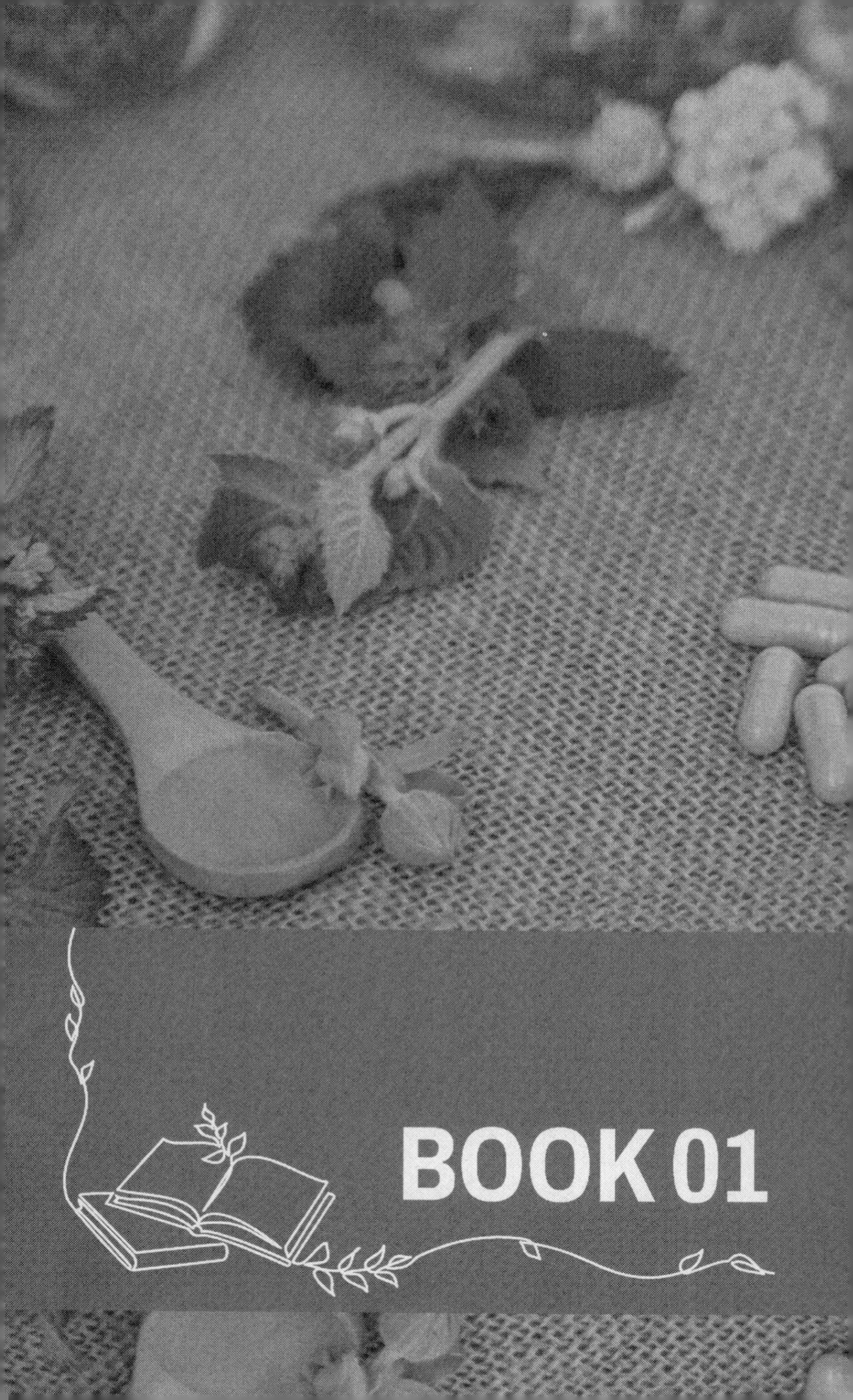
BOOK 01

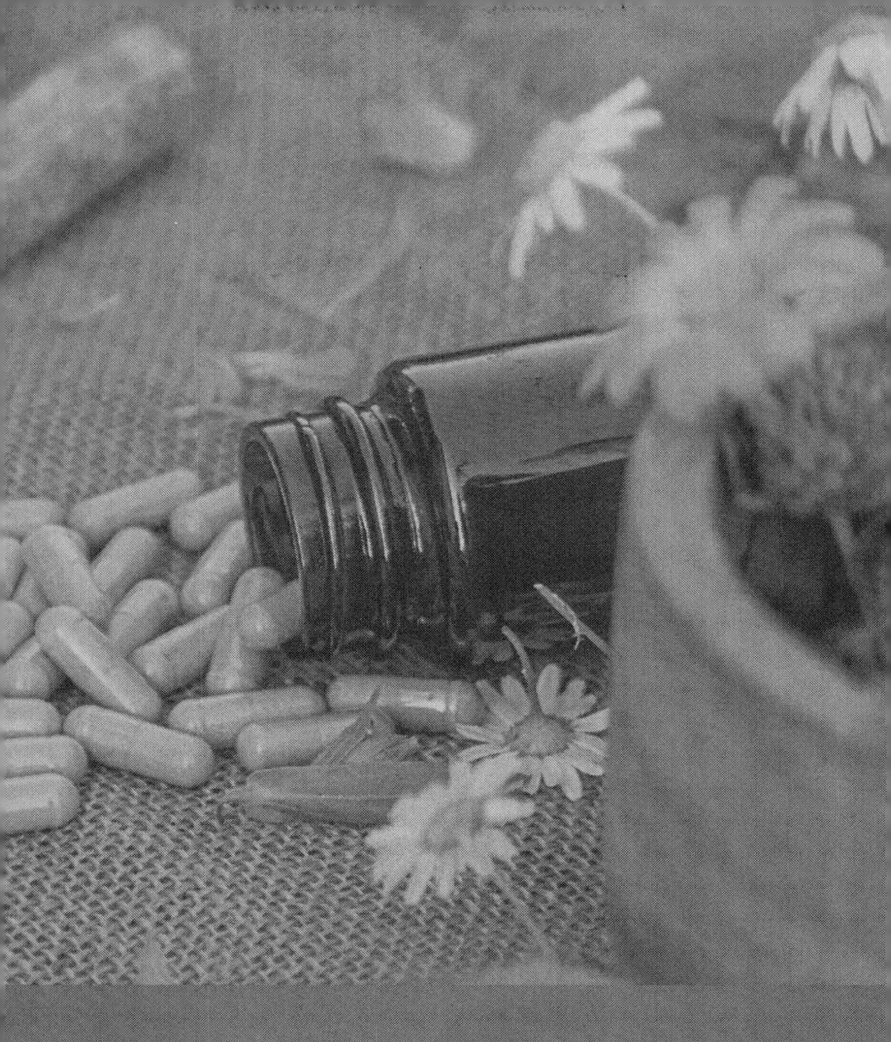

Holistic Cures and Natural Antibiotics for Complete Healing

CHAPTER 01

Foundations of Herbal Healing and Safety

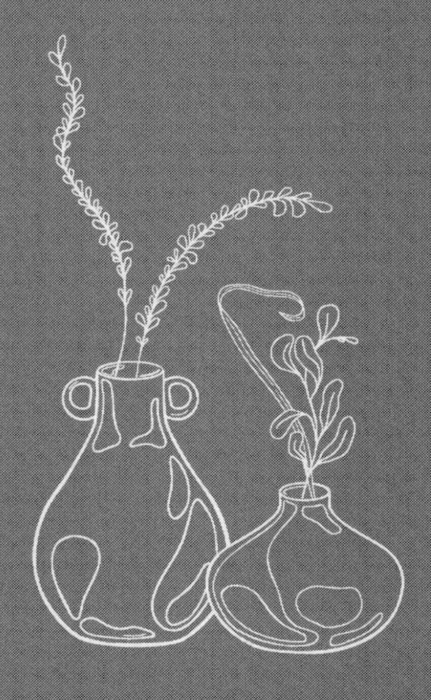

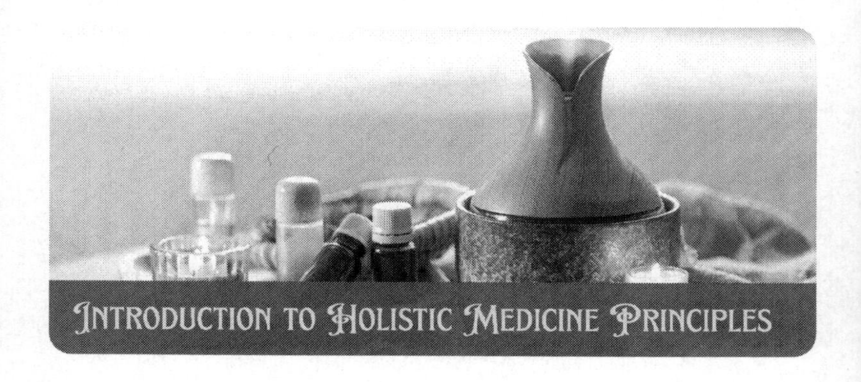

Introduction to Holistic Medicine Principles

At its core, holistic medicine recognizes that health is more than the absence of disease; it's a state of complete physical, mental, and spiritual well-being. Unlike conventional medicine, which often focuses only on treating specific symptoms, holistic medicine emphasizes the importance of treating the whole person. By considering the interconnectedness of the body, mind, and spirit, holistic practitioners aim to address the root causes of illness rather than simply alleviating symptoms. This approach allows for a deeper, more sustainable path to wellness by recognizing the body's innate ability to heal itself when properly supported.

In holistic medicine, every aspect of a person's life-from diet and sleep to emotional health and lifestyle choices-plays a role in their overall well-being. Rather than viewing the body as a collection of isolated systems, holistic medicine sees it as a cohesive, interconnected whole. Practitioners believe that imbalances in one area of life can lead to physical ailments elsewhere. For example, chronic stress can not only affect mental health, but also weaken the immune system, making the body more susceptible to infection. The goal of holistic medicine is to identify and restore balance within these systems so that the body can function optimally.

Another fundamental tenet of holistic medicine is prevention. While many conventional treatments focus on treating symptoms after they occur, holistic approaches emphasize prevention through lifestyle adjustments, diet, and mindfulness practices. Prevention is seen as the most effective path to long-term health, and individuals are empowered to make choices that support their wellness journey. Holistic practitioners encourage self-awareness and regular assessment of one's health, as early intervention can often prevent more serious conditions from developing.

Herbal medicine fits seamlessly into the holistic approach. One of the oldest healing traditions, it uses plants and plant-derived substances to support the body's natural processes. Herbs work with the body's systems to gently promote healing and restore balance. Unlike many synthetic drugs, which can disrupt or overwhelm the body's natural rhythms, herbs tend to work in harmony with these processes. For example, chamomile can calm the nervous system without the sedative side effects of pharmaceutical sleep aids, while ginger aids digestion by stimulating the body's own digestive enzymes.

A key component of holistic herbalism is understanding the "energetics" of both plants and people. In herbal medicine, each plant has specific qualities - such as warming, cooling, moisturizing, or drying - that affect how it interacts with the body. Similarly, people have different constitutions or natural tendencies that affect their health. A person with a "cold" constitution might benefit from "warming" herbs such as ginger or cinnamon, while a person with a "hot" constitution might find balance in "cooling" herbs such as peppermint. By matching herbs to a person's constitution, holistic herbalism can provide personalized, effective support.

The popularity of holistic practices, including herbal medicine, has grown in recent years as individuals seek gentler alternatives to pharmaceuticals. However, it's important to recognize that holistic medicine is not an all-or-nothing approach. Integrative medicine, which combines conventional treatments with holistic practices, allows people to benefit from both. Many find that herbal remedies can complement traditional care, providing relief and support without the side effects often associated with pharmaceuticals.

This book offers a wide range of remedies and techniques rooted in holistic principles. Whether for respiratory support, digestive health, or immune function, the goal is to help readers build a toolkit of natural options to support their health. These remedies work not only to treat ailments as they arise, but also to promote a balanced, resilient state of well-being.

Holistic medicine ultimately invites each person to take an active role in their health by making conscious choices that align with their body's needs and support them with natural resources. As you explore the remedies and techniques in this book, keep in mind the core principles of holistic wellness: balance, prevention, and treating the whole self. These principles will guide you as you begin to integrate natural practices into your daily life, creating a foundation of wellness that goes beyond the immediate treatment of symptoms.

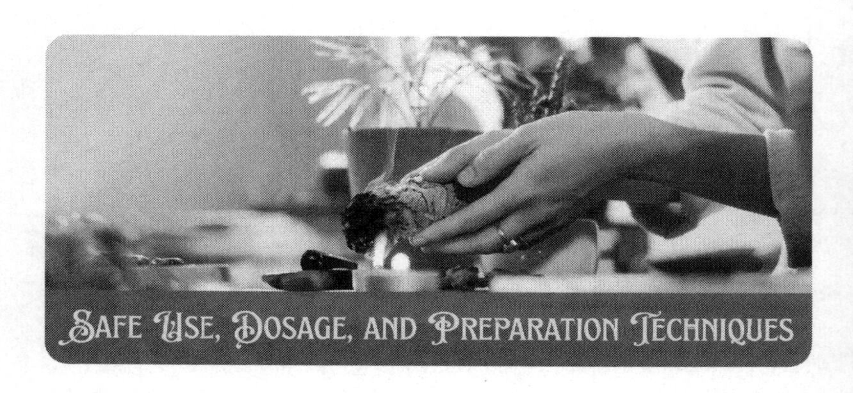

Safe Use, Dosage, and Preparation Techniques

When it comes to incorporating herbal remedies into your health routine, safety is paramount. While herbal medicine is generally gentle and well-tolerated, herbs can be powerful and must be used responsibly to maximize benefits and minimize risks. Understanding the principles of safe use, proper dosage, and proper preparation techniques is essential. This section will guide you through these essential aspects to ensure that your experience with herbal remedies is both effective and safe.

The Importance of Accurate Dosage

As with conventional medications, dosage is important with herbal remedies. While herbs may seem harmless, taking the wrong dose can render them ineffective or, in some cases, cause adverse effects. The appropriate dosage varies widely depending on factors such as the herb itself, a person's age, body weight, constitution, and any underlying health conditions.

Adult Dosages: Herbal dosages for adults are typically calculated based on average body weight, usually around 150 pounds. A common guideline for tinctures, for example, is 1-2 tablespoons (about 20-40 drops) one to three times a day. For dried herbs used in teas or capsules, the standard dose may be 1 to 3 grams per day, divided into smaller doses.

Adaptations for children: Children require much smaller doses, often calculated as a fraction of the adult dose based on their weight. Young's Rule" or "Clark's Rule" are commonly used formulas to determine appropriate pediatric dosages. Always use caution when administering herbs to children and consult a healthcare professional if in doubt.

Use cautiously in the elderly: Older adults may have altered metabolism and organ function, requiring lower doses and careful monitoring. Starting with a low dose and adjusting as needed is a prudent approach.

Starting with a minimal dose and gradually increasing it allows you to observe how your body responds. This practice, known as "titration," helps determine the most effective and safe dose. Always listen to your body's feedback and if you experience any adverse effects, discontinue use and seek medical advice.

Understanding Preparation Methods

The way herbs are prepared affects their potency, effectiveness, and safety. Different methods of preparation extract different compounds from the plant, so it is important to choose the right technique based on your goals.

Infusions: Infusions are made by steeping delicate plant parts, such as leaves and flowers, in hot water. This method is ideal for extracting vitamins, minerals, and aromatic compounds. Use 1-2 teaspoons of dried herbs per cup of boiling water and steep for 10-15 minutes. Infusions are perfect for calming herbs like chamomile or nutrient-rich options like stinging nettle.

Decoctions: Decoctions are more appropriate for tougher plant materials such as roots, bark, and seeds. To make a decoction, simmer the herb in water for 20-30 minutes to extract the beneficial compounds. For example, boiling ginger root helps release its warming, anti-inflammatory properties.

Tinctures: Tinctures are concentrated liquid extracts made by soaking herbs in alcohol or glycerin. Alcohol-based tinctures are potent and have a long shelf life, but glycerin-based tinctures are a gentler, non-alcoholic alternative, ideal for children or those who avoid alcohol. The standard ratio for making tinctures is one part herb to five parts alcohol or glycerin, steeped for four to six weeks.

Salves and ointments: These are made by infusing oils with herbs and combining them with beeswax to create a topical application. Salves are great for treating skin conditions or muscle aches. For example, marigold oil mixed with beeswax can be used to make a soothing salve for dry, irritated skin.

Poultices and compresses: A poultice is a paste of herbs applied directly to the skin, while a compress is a cloth soaked in a strong herbal infusion. These methods are effective for treating bruises, wounds, or inflammation. For example, a comfrey poultice can help relieve sprains and promote healing.

Choosing the appropriate method of preparation is critical to achieving the desired therapeutic effect. Teas and tinctures are generally more appropriate for internal use, while compresses and ointments are ideal for external application.

Essential Safety Precautions

Although herbs are natural, they should be used with the same caution as any other medication. Here are some important safety precautions to keep in mind:

Be aware of potential allergies: Before using a new herb, especially in large amounts, consider doing a patch test or consuming a small amount to check for allergic reactions. Skin rashes, itching, or digestive upset are signs of a possible allergy.

Understand herb-drug interactions: Some herbs may interact with medications. For example, St. John's wort is known to interfere with antidepressants, birth control pills, and blood thinners. Always consult a healthcare provider if you are taking prescription medications or have a chronic medical condition.

Pregnancy and lactation considerations: Pregnant and breastfeeding women should use extra caution with herbal remedies because some herbs may interfere with pregnancy or be harmful to a developing baby. Herbs such as blue cohosh, pennyroyal, and goldenseal are generally not recommended during pregnancy.

Know the difference between culinary and medicinal use: Many herbs that are safe in culinary amounts, such as nutmeg or sage, can have potent effects when used in higher, medicinal doses. It's important to use herbs responsibly and to understand when they transition from food to medicine.

Monitor for side effects: Common side effects of herbs may include digestive upset, skin irritation, or mild headache. If you experience severe or persistent symptoms, stop using the herb and seek medical attention.

Storage Tips to Maintain Potency

Proper storage is essential to keeping your herbs fresh and potent. Herbs can lose their potency when exposed to light, heat, or moisture. Here's how to ensure that your herbal preparations maintain their quality:

Dried herbs: Store dried herbs in airtight containers, preferably glass jars, in a cool, dark place. Avoid plastic containers, which can degrade over time and leach chemicals into the herbs. Well stored dried herbs can maintain their potency for up to a year.

Tinctures and oils: Store tinctures in dark glass bottles to protect them from light. Essential oils and infused oils should be stored in a cool, dark place to extend their shelf life. Properly stored tinctures can last several years, while oils typically remain potent for up to six months to a year.

Ointments and balms: These should be stored in airtight containers away from heat and sunlight. Be sure to label each preparation with the date it was made so you'll know when it's time to make a fresh batch.

General Guidelines for Safe Herbal Practice

Label everything clearly: Each herbal preparation should be labeled with the name of the herb, the date of preparation, and any important directions for use. This practice reduces the risk of inadvertent misuse.

Practice hygiene: Always wash your hands and use clean utensils when preparing herbal remedies. Cross-contamination can affect the purity and safety of your preparations.

Consult a professional: If you're ever unsure about the safety of an herb or its interaction with medications, seek the advice of a trained herbalist or healthcare provider.

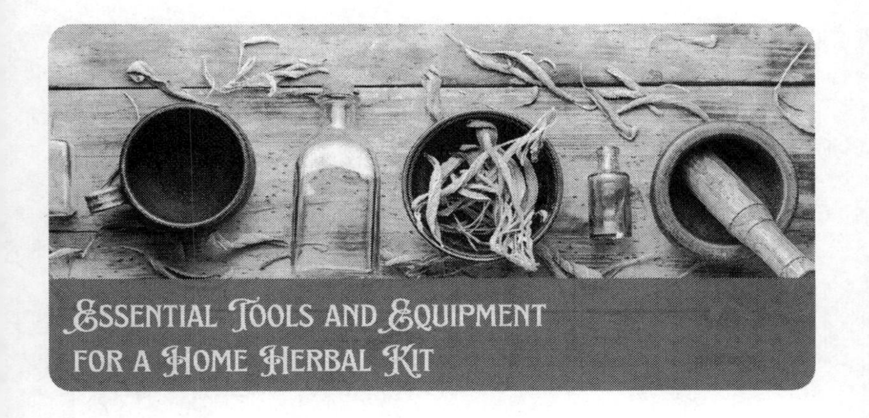

Essential Tools and Equipment for a Home Herbal Kit

Creating an effective home herbal kit is a fundamental step for anyone committed to natural healing. With the right tools and equipment, preparing and storing your herbal remedies becomes a streamlined and efficient process.

An organized and well-stocked herbal kit ensures that you have everything you need at your fingertips, from making simple teas to creating potent ointments and tinctures. This section will guide you through the essential items needed to create a reliable and functional herbal kit, setting you up for a safe and successful herbal practice.

1. Storage Containers and Glass Jars

Proper storage is critical to maintaining the potency and freshness of your herbs. Herbs, tinctures, and ointments are best stored in glass containers, which are non-reactive and protect the contents from external contaminants.

Glass jars: Use airtight glass jars for dried herbs. Dark glass, such as amber or cobalt blue, is ideal because it protects the herbs from sunlight, which can degrade their active compounds. Choose different sizes to accommodate different amounts of herbs.

Dropper Bottles: Essential for storing tinctures and liquid extracts, dropper bottles allow for precise dosing and are easy to label. These come in 1-2 ounce sizes and are typically made of dark glass to preserve the quality of the liquid.

Salve jars: Metal jars or small glass jars with secure lids are perfect for homemade salves, ointments, and balms. These containers are both convenient and portable, making them ideal for use on the go.

2. Measuring Tools for Precision

Accurate measurements are critical in herbal medicine to ensure the proper dosage and potency of your preparations.

Digital Weighing Scale: A small, accurate digital scale is essential for measuring dried herbs. It should be sensitive enough to measure small amounts in grams or ounces, as many herbal recipes call for exact quantities.

Measuring spoons and cups: A standard set of measuring spoons and cups ensures consistency when preparing teas, infusions, or oil blends. Choose durable, easy-to-clean tools, and consider a separate set for herbal work to avoid cross-contamination with kitchen items.

3. Tools for Grinding and Mixing

Some herbs require grinding or mixing before use, so a few basic tools are essential.

Mortar and pestle: A mortar and pestle are classic tools for grinding herbs into powders or mixing different ingredients. Marble or ceramic versions are ideal because they are nonporous and won't absorb oils or moisture from the herbs.

Herb grinder: For tougher plant materials, a special herb grinder (similar to a coffee grinder) can save time and effort. Be sure to clean it thoroughly between uses to prevent contamination.

4. Strainers and Filtering Tools

Filtering is a key step in herbal preparation, especially when making teas, tinctures, and infused oils.

Fine mesh strainer: A stainless steel fine mesh strainer is great for filtering infusions and decoctions. It traps small particles, leaving you with a smooth liquid.

Cheesecloth or muslin bags: These are versatile tools for straining and infusing herbs. Cheesecloth can be used to strain large amounts of liquid, while muslin bags are great for making herbal bath soaks or large infusions.

5. Funnels for Easy Pouring

A set of funnels makes transferring liquid preparations to storage containers much easier and cleaner.

Glass or stainless steel funnels: These materials are preferred for their durability and ease of cleaning. Having a few different sizes can be helpful when dealing with different container openings.

6. Double Boiler for Infused Oils and Salves

A double boiler is necessary for gently heating herbs and oils, especially when making salves or infused oils. Direct heat can destroy beneficial compounds, so a double boiler allows for even, controlled heating.

Heat-resistant glass or stainless steel: Use materials that are non-reactive and won't affect the quality of the oils or herbs. If you don't have a special double boiler, you can improvise with a heatproof bowl over a pot of simmering water.

7. Mixing Bowls and Utensils

Having a variety of mixing bowls and utensils designated for herbal preparations will make your work easier and more organized.

Glass or ceramic bowls: Use non-reactive bowls for mixing herbs, as they won't leach chemicals or change the properties of your preparations.

Wooden or silicone utensils: These are gentle on your mixing bowls and prevent reactions with herbs, especially when you're working with acidic ingredients.

8. Labeling Supplies for Organization

Clear labeling is an important part of herbal practice, helping you keep track of your remedies and avoid confusion.

Waterproof labels: Choose labels that can withstand exposure to moisture and oil. Each label should include the name of the herb, the date of preparation, and any special instructions or dosage recommendations.

Permanent markers: Fine-tip, oil-resistant markers are best for writing on labels to ensure information remains legible over time.

9. Spray Bottles for Herbal Mists and Sprays

Spray bottles are useful for making herbal mists, room sprays, or topical skin applications.

Glass spray bottles: Choose dark glass bottles to protect delicate ingredients from light. They are perfect for storing and using homemade facial mists, air fresheners, or herbal insect repellents.

10. Notebooks for Documentation

Keeping a detailed record of your herbal preparations is invaluable for tracking their effectiveness and refining your methods.

Herbal Journal: Use a special notebook to document your recipes, observations, and adjustments. Record the herbs used, preparation methods, and any effects or feedback. This practice not only helps you improve your herbal skills, but also serves as a reference for future use.

Setting Up Your Home Herbal Space

Organize your herbal tools and supplies in a dedicated space, such as a kitchen cabinet or small shelf unit. Group items by function: storage containers together, mixing tools in one area, and preparation equipment in another. Keeping everything organized and easily accessible will make the herbal preparation process smoother and more enjoyable.

By assembling a well-stocked and organized herbal kit, you're setting yourself up for success in your natural healing journey. These tools and equipment will make your herbal practice efficient, safe, and effective, allowing you to create remedies with confidence and precision.

CHAPTER 2

Natural Antibiotics and Antimicrobials

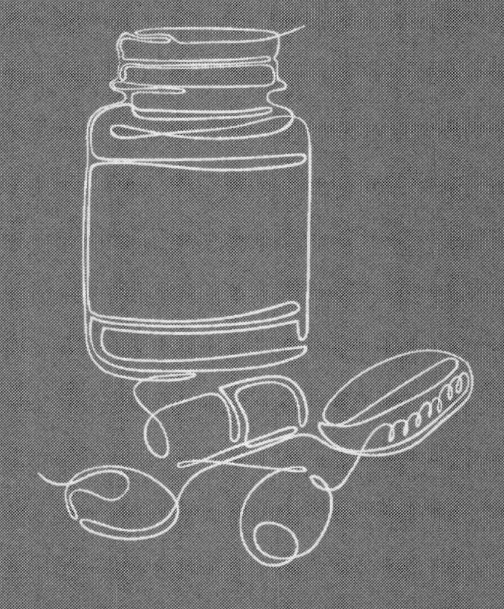

The overuse of synthetic antibiotics in modern healthcare has led to widespread concerns about antibiotic resistance and the search for safer, more sustainable alternatives. While conventional antibiotics have saved countless lives, they often come with side effects and can disrupt the body's natural microbiome. This chapter focuses on natural antibiotics and antimicrobial herbs, highlighting their traditional uses, scientific support, and practical applications. By understanding how these natural agents work, you can incorporate them into your health routine to fight infections and support overall wellness safely and effectively.

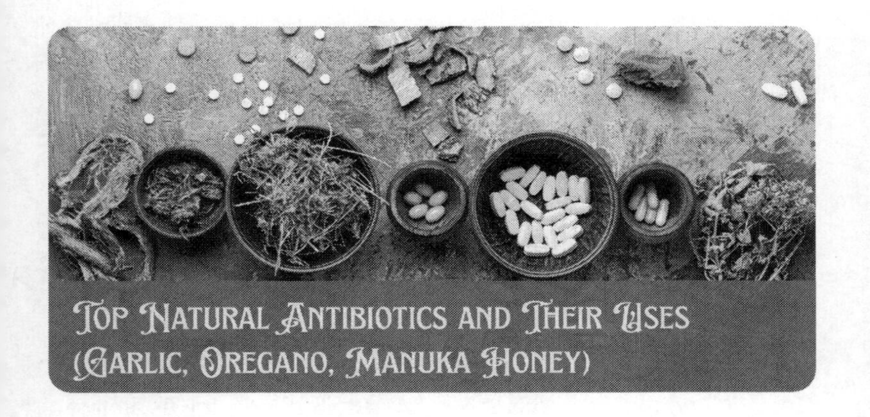

Top Natural Antibiotics and Their Uses (Garlic, Oregano, Manuka Honey)

Nature has provided us with a variety of powerful antimicrobial agents that have been used for centuries to fight infections and support the body's immune defenses. Among the most well-known and scientifically validated are garlic, oregano, and Manuka honey. These natural antibiotics are valued not only for their effectiveness, but also for their relative gentleness on the body compared to synthetic antibiotics.

1. Garlic (Allium sativum)

Garlic has been revered as a medicinal powerhouse for thousands of years. Ancient civilizations, including the Egyptians and Greeks, used garlic for its healing properties, and modern research continues to validate its effectiveness. The key component in garlic responsible for its potent antimicrobial activity is allicin, a sulfur-containing compound that is released when garlic is crushed or chopped.

Antibacterial properties: Garlic has been shown to fight a wide range of bacteria, including antibiotic-resistant strains such as MRSA (methicillin-resistant Staphylococcus aureus). It disrupts the cell walls of bacteria, preventing them from thriving and spreading. Research also suggests that garlic may be effective against Helicobacter pylori, a bacteria associated with stomach ulcers.

Antiviral and antifungal effects: In addition to its antibacterial properties, garlic has antiviral effects, making it a useful remedy during cold and flu season. It can also help fight fungal infections such as candida by inhibiting the growth of yeast.

Practical applications: To take advantage of garlic's antibiotic power, it's best to eat it raw, as cooking can reduce the allicin content. Crushing a clove and letting it sit for 10 minutes before eating helps activate the allicin. Garlic-infused oil can also be applied topically for infections, although care should be taken not to use it on sensitive or damaged skin.

2. Oregano (Origanum vulgare)

Oregano, a popular culinary herb, also holds a place in the natural medicine cabinet for its potent antimicrobial properties. The essential oil extracted from oregano leaves is particularly potent thanks to compounds such as carvacrol and thymol, both of which have been extensively studied for their antibacterial and antifungal effects.

Antibacterial action: Oregano oil is effective against a number of bacteria, including Staphylococcus and E. coli. Its compounds work by disrupting the cell membranes of bacteria, making it difficult for them to survive. Studies have also shown that oregano oil can inhibit the growth of certain foodborne pathogens, making it a valuable food safety tool.

Antifungal and antiparasitic properties: Beyond bacteria, oregano oil is a well-known antifungal agent, often used to treat conditions such as athlete's foot and candida overgrowth. It also has antiparasitic properties that can be beneficial for gastrointestinal health.

Practical Uses: Oregano oil is incredibly potent and should always be diluted before use. For internal use, mix a drop of oregano oil with a carrier oil, such as olive or coconut oil, and consume in small amounts. For topical use, dilute the oil and apply to affected areas, avoiding mucous membranes and sensitive skin.

3. Manuka Honey

Manuka honey, produced by bees pollinating the Manuka bush (Leptospermum scoparium) in New Zealand, is renowned for its extraordinary healing properties. Unlike regular honey, Manuka honey contains Methylglyoxal (MGO), a compound that gives it powerful antimicrobial activity. The unique properties of Manuka Honey have made it the subject of extensive research, particularly in wound care and infection prevention.

Antibacterial Potency: Manuka Honey has been shown to inhibit a wide range of bacteria, including Staphylococcus aureus and Streptococcus pyogenes. It creates an inhospitable environment for bacteria by drawing moisture from bacterial cells, effectively dehydrating and killing them. Its use in hospitals to treat wounds and burns demonstrates its efficacy and safety.

Wound healing and anti-inflammatory effects: One of the outstanding benefits of Manuka Honey is its ability to promote wound healing and reduce inflammation. It not only fights infection, but also accelerates tissue regeneration and soothes irritation.

Practical applications: Manuka Honey can be applied directly to wounds and skin infections to aid healing. For sore throats and internal infections it can be taken by the spoonful or added to herbal teas. It's important to choose high quality, medical grade Manuka Honey, as not all products labeled "Manuka" contain significant levels of MGO.

How to Use These Natural Antibiotics Safely

While garlic, oregano, and Manuka honey are effective and generally well tolerated, it's important to use them with caution:

Garlic: High doses of garlic may cause gastrointestinal upset or interact with blood-thinning medications. Always start with small amounts and monitor for adverse effects.

Oregano Oil: This oil is highly concentrated and may be irritating to the skin and mucous membranes if not properly diluted. Avoid prolonged use without consulting a healthcare professional.

Manuka Honey: Although safe for most people, people with diabetes should use Manuka Honey with caution due to its sugar content. In addition, infants under one year of age should not consume honey of any kind due to the risk of botulism.

These natural antibiotics can be a powerful part of your health toolbox. By understanding their unique properties and knowing how to use them properly, you can tap into nature's healing potential and support your body's defenses in a safe and effective way. In the next section, we'll explore powerful antifungal and antiviral herbs that further enhance our natural medicine arsenal.

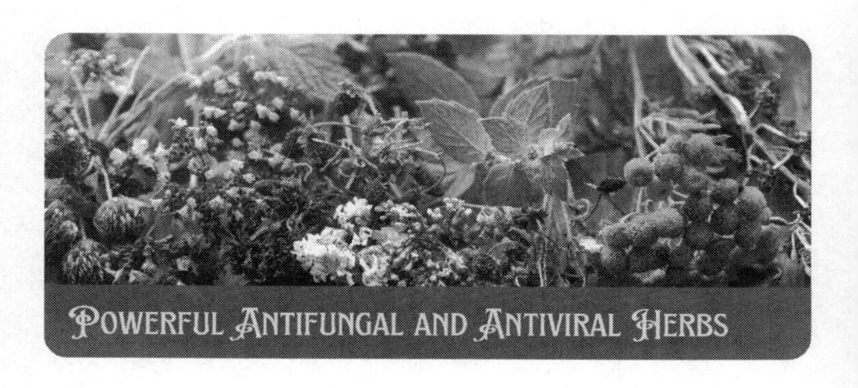

Powerful Antifungal and Antiviral Herbs

In addition to natural antibiotics, there are a variety of herbs with potent antifungal and antiviral properties that have been used for centuries to combat infections and support immune health. These herbs offer a natural way to manage fungal infections, such as athlete's foot or yeast overgrowth, as well as viral illnesses like the common cold and flu. Understanding the unique benefits of these powerful herbs allows you to choose the right remedy for specific health concerns.

Echinacea (Echinacea purpurea and Echinacea angustifolia)

Echinacea is a well-known herb in the world of natural medicine, praised for its immune-boosting and antiviral effects. Often used at the onset of colds and flu, echinacea contains compounds that stimulate the body's natural defenses and increase the activity of white blood cells that fight off infection. Studies have shown that echinacea can reduce the severity and duration of respiratory infections, making it a valuable ally during cold and flu season. It is most effective when taken at the first sign of illness and can be taken as a tea, tincture, or capsule.

Elderberry (Sambucus nigra)

Elderberry has long been used to fight off viral infections. Rich in antioxidants and flavonoids, elderberries have been shown to inhibit the replication of viruses, especially those responsible for colds and flu. Elderberry syrup is a popular remedy for reducing flu symptoms, including fever, cough, and body aches. Elderberry's anti-inflammatory properties also help soothe irritated airways. This herb is commonly used in syrups, gums, and teas and is well tolerated by most people. However, raw elderberries should never be consumed as they contain compounds that can cause nausea and vomiting if not properly cooked.

Pau d'Arco (Tabebuia impetiginosa)

Pau d'Arco, a bark extract from the Lapacho tree native to South America, is a potent antifungal herb with a long history of use among indigenous populations. It contains naphthoquinones, compounds known for their antifungal and immune-boosting properties. Pau d'arco is often used to treat fungal infections such as candida overgrowth, athlete's foot, and toenail fungus. It can be prepared as a tea or taken in capsule form. However, caution should be exercised when using pau d'arco in large doses or for prolonged periods, as it may cause gastrointestinal upset in some people.

Lemon Balm (Melissa officinalis)

Lemon balm is a gentle yet effective antiviral herb often used to calm the nervous system and fight viral infections. It has been studied for its ability to fight the herpes simplex virus (HSV) and is often used as a topical remedy to reduce the severity and duration of cold sores. Internally, lemon balm can be taken as a tea to relieve stress, anxiety, and viral infections such as the common cold. Its calming properties make it a versatile herb that provides both antiviral and stress-relieving benefits.

Tea Tree Oil (Melaleuca alternifolia)

Tea tree oil is a potent antifungal and antiviral essential oil, widely recognized for its use in treating skin infections, fungal overgrowth, and respiratory problems. It contains terpinen-4-ol, a compound that gives it strong antimicrobial activity. Tea tree oil is often used topically to treat athlete's foot, ringworm, and warts, but it should never be ingested due to its potency and risk of toxicity. When using tea tree oil, it is important to dilute it with a carrier oil to prevent skin irritation. A few drops mixed with coconut oil can be an effective remedy for fungal and viral skin conditions.

These antifungal and antiviral herbs provide a natural and effective way to support your immune system and fight infections. As with all herbal treatments, understanding the properties and appropriate use of each herb will ensure safe and effective results.

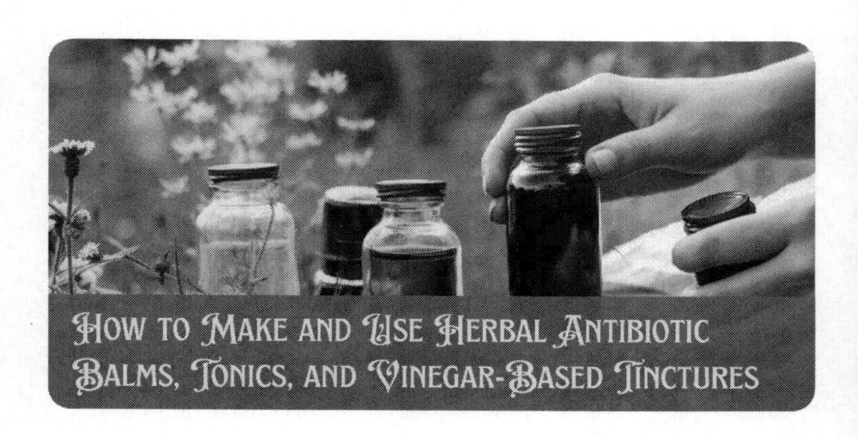

Making your own herbal remedies at home is a rewarding and empowering way to take control of your health. Herbal balms, tonics, and vinegar-based tinctures are versatile preparations that can be used to support the immune system, soothe skin infections, and fight bacterial and viral threats. This section will guide you through the basics of making these natural remedies, offering practical techniques and safety tips.

Herbal Antibiotic Balms

Herbal balms are ointments made by infusing oils with antibacterial herbs and then solidifying the mixture with beeswax. These balms can be applied topically to cuts, scrapes, burns, and insect bites to prevent infection and promote healing. Popular herbs for antibiotic balms include marigold, comfrey, and St. John's wort, all known for their antimicrobial and soothing properties.

To make a simple herbal antibiotic balm:

- **Infuse the oil:** Combine dried herbs (such as marigold and comfrey) with olive oil in a glass jar. Seal the jar and place in a warm, sunny spot for 2-4 weeks, shaking daily to release the herbs' beneficial compounds. Alternatively, you can use a double boiler to gently heat the herbs and oil for a few hours.
- **Strain the oil:** Once infused, strain the oil through a fine mesh sieve or cheesecloth to remove all plant material.
- **Prepare the balm:** Melt the beeswax in a double boiler, then stir in the infused oil. The typical ratio is 1 ounce of beeswax to 8 ounces of oil. Pour the mixture into small cans or glass jars and allow to cool and solidify. Label the containers and store in a cool, dark place.

Immune-Boosting Tonics

Herbal tonics are liquid preparations designed to strengthen the body's defenses and promote overall health. Fire Cider is a popular immune-boosting tonic made with vinegar and a blend of antimicrobial herbs and spices such as garlic, ginger, horseradish, and cayenne pepper. The ingredients are infused in apple cider vinegar, which helps extract the beneficial compounds from the herbs and also acts as a natural preservative.

To make a basic fire cider:

- **Combine ingredients:** In a large glass jar, add minced garlic, grated ginger, diced horseradish root, and a few slices of hot pepper. Pour raw apple cider vinegar over the herbs until they are completely submerged.
- **Infuse:** Seal the jar with a non-metallic lid (vinegar can corrode metal) and let the mixture sit at room temperature for 4-6 weeks. Shake the jar daily to aid in the infusion process.

- **Strain and store:** At the end of the infusion period, strain the liquid and discard the solids. Store the fire cider in a glass bottle and take 1-2 tablespoons daily as an immune booster, especially during cold and flu season.

Vinegar-Based Tinctures

Vinegar-based tinctures are a great alcohol-free alternative for extracting the medicinal properties of herbs. Apple cider vinegar is often used because it has additional health benefits and is easily absorbed by the body. Herbs such as thyme, rosemary, and oregano are excellent choices for making antimicrobial tinctures.

To prepare a vinegar-based tincture:

- **Fill a jar with herbs:** Place fresh or dried herbs in a glass jar, filling it about halfway. Pour apple cider vinegar over the herbs, making sure they are completely covered.
- **Infuse the tincture:** Seal the jar and store in a cool, dark place for 3-4 weeks, shaking daily to aid in the extraction process.
- **Strain and use:** Strain the tincture through cheesecloth and transfer the liquid to a dropper bottle. Vinegar-based tinctures can be taken in small doses (1-2 teaspoons) or added to salads and meals for a health boost.

Making herbal balms, tonics, and tinctures takes patience and attention to detail, but the results are effective and empowering. These natural preparations allow you to harness the healing power of herbs in a way that is both practical and accessible, offering safe and gentle support for your health.

CHAPTER 3

Holistic Remedies for Common Health Concerns

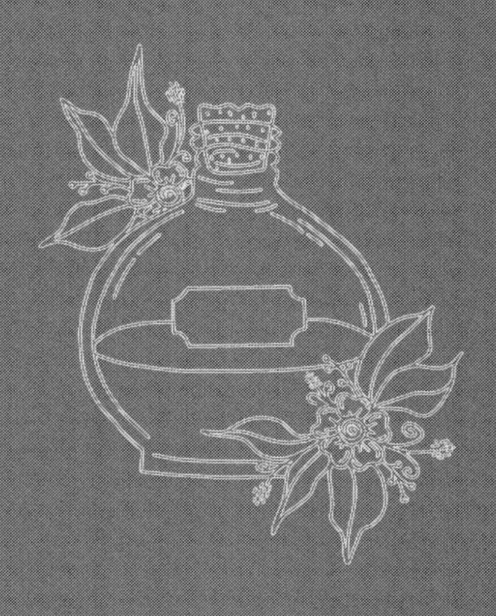

Common health problems such as respiratory infections, digestive disorders, and skin irritations can disrupt daily life and reduce overall well-being. Instead of turning to conventional medicine, many people are turning to holistic remedies for gentle yet effective relief. By harnessing the natural properties of herbs, we can support the body's natural healing processes while minimizing the side effects often associated with pharmaceuticals. This chapter explores holistic approaches to treating common ailments, with an emphasis on safety, efficacy, and practical application.

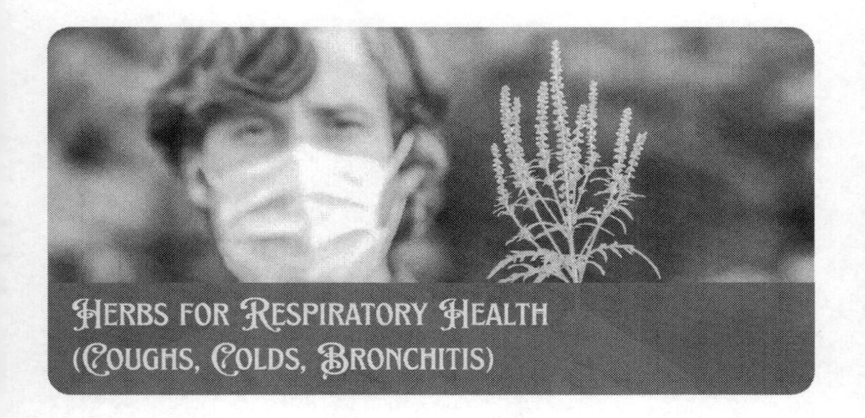

Herbs for Respiratory Health (Coughs, Colds, Bronchitis)

Respiratory health is a fundamental aspect of overall well-being. The respiratory system is constantly exposed to the outside environment, making it susceptible to infections, allergens, and irritants. Herbs have long been used to relieve symptoms such as coughing, congestion, and bronchial inflammation, supporting respiratory function and helping to clear the airways. This section explores some of the most effective herbs for respiratory health and how to use them safely.

Mullein (Verbascum thapsus)

Mullein is a classic respiratory herb known for its soothing and anti-inflammatory properties. The leaves and flowers of the mullein plant have been used for centuries to treat coughs, colds, and bronchitis. Mullein acts as an expectorant, helping to loosen and expel mucus from the lungs, making it easier to breathe. It also has a demulcent effect, which means it coats and soothes irritated mucous membranes in the throat and lungs.

How to use: Mullein can be made into a tea by steeping the dried leaves in hot water for 10-15 minutes. Strain the tea carefully through a fine-mesh strainer or cheesecloth to remove any small hairs from the plant, which can be irritating if ingested. Drinking mullein tea a few times a day may help relieve coughs and congestion. It is gentle and safe for most people, but always consult a healthcare professional if you are pregnant or taking any medications.

Thyme (Thymus vulgaris)

Thyme is a powerful antimicrobial and antiviral herb, making it an excellent remedy for respiratory infections. It is rich in thymol, a compound that has been shown to help fight respiratory pathogens and reduce inflammation. Thyme also has expectorant properties that help clear mucus from the lungs, making it especially useful for conditions such as bronchitis and chronic cough.

How to use: Thyme can be prepared as a tea or used in steam inhalations. To make thyme tea, steep 1-2 teaspoons of dried thyme in a cup of boiling water for 10 minutes, then strain and drink. For a steam inhalation, add a few sprigs of fresh thyme or a few drops of thyme essential oil to a bowl of hot water, cover your head with a towel, and inhale the steam for several minutes. This helps open the airways and relieve congestion.

Eucalyptus (Eucalyptus globulus)

Eucalyptus is known for its ability to clear the sinuses and promote easy breathing. The essential oil of eucalyptus contains eucalyptol (1,8-cineol), which has been studied for its effectiveness in reducing nasal congestion and opening the bronchial tubes. Eucalyptus also has antibacterial and anti-inflammatory properties, making it a popular choice for respiratory problems.

How to use: Eucalyptus essential oil should never be ingested, but can be used in steam inhalations or diluted and applied topically. For a steam inhalation, add 2-3 drops of eucalyptus oil to a bowl of hot water, cover your head with a towel, and inhale the steam for several minutes. For topical application, dilute eucalyptus oil with a carrier oil, such as coconut or olive oil, and rub it on the chest to relieve congestion. Avoid using eucalyptus oil on young children or people with asthma, as it can sometimes cause bronchial spasms.

Licorice Root (Glycyrrhiza glabra)

Licorice root is a versatile herb with both anti-inflammatory and soothing properties, making it beneficial for respiratory health. It acts as an expectorant, helping to clear mucus from the airways, and also soothes sore throats and irritated respiratory tissues. However, due to its effect on cortisol and blood pressure, licorice root should be used with caution, especially by individuals with hypertension or pregnant women.

How to use: Licorice root can be consumed as a tea by boiling the dried root in water for 10-15 minutes. Drink 1-2 cups daily to soothe the throat and reduce coughing. For a sore throat, licorice root tea can also be used as a gargle.

Peppermint (Mentha piperita)

Peppermint is known for its refreshing scent and ability to relieve congestion. The main active ingredient, menthol, acts as a natural decongestant, helping to break up mucus and open the nasal passages. Peppermint also has antispasmodic properties that can help relax the muscles of the respiratory tract, making it easier to breathe.

How to use: Peppermint tea is an easy way to relieve congestion and soothe the throat. Steep fresh or dried peppermint leaves in hot water for 5-10 minutes, strain, and drink. Peppermint essential oil can also be used in steam inhalations or diluted with a carrier oil and applied to the chest. As with eucalyptus, avoid using peppermint oil on young children.

These herbs provide natural, effective support for respiratory health. By understanding how to use them properly, you can manage symptoms such as coughs, congestion, and bronchial irritation with confidence. In the following sections, we'll explore holistic remedies for digestive and skin health to ensure you have a well-rounded approach to managing common health concerns.

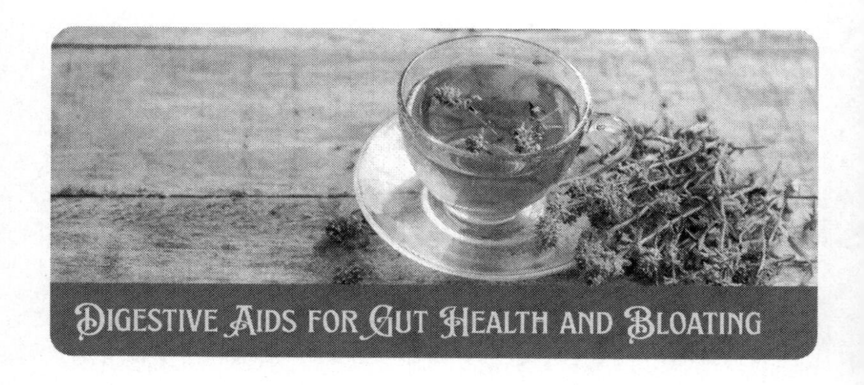

Digestive Aids for Gut Health and Bloating

Digestive discomfort and bloating are common problems that can significantly impact daily well-being. From occasional indigestion to chronic gastrointestinal conditions, these disorders can interfere with the body's ability to absorb nutrients and eliminate waste. Fortunately, there are several herbs known for their ability to soothe the digestive tract, reduce bloating, and promote overall gut health. These natural remedies not only provide relief from discomfort, but also help restore balance to the digestive system, ensuring optimal function.

Ginger (Zingiber officinale)

Ginger has been used for centuries to aid digestion and relieve nausea. Its active constituents, gingerols and shogaols, have anti-inflammatory and antispasmodic properties that relax gastrointestinal muscles, making it easier for the body to pass food and gas. Ginger is particularly effective for bloating, indigestion, and motion sickness.

How to use: Ginger tea is a simple and effective remedy for digestive problems. Slice fresh ginger root and steep in hot water for 10-15 minutes. Add honey if desired. Drinking ginger tea before meals can stimulate digestive enzymes and help prevent gas. Ginger can also be taken in capsule form or added to meals as a flavorful digestive aid.

Peppermint (Mentha piperita)

Peppermint is widely known for its ability to relieve gas and support digestive health. The menthol in peppermint has a soothing effect on the muscles of the gastrointestinal tract, helping to relieve gas and cramping. Peppermint oil in particular has been shown to be effective in treating symptoms of irritable bowel syndrome (IBS), such as abdominal pain and bloating.

How to use: Peppermint tea is a popular choice for soothing indigestion. Steep fresh or dried peppermint leaves in hot water for 5-10 minutes and drink after meals. Peppermint oil capsules can also be used, but they should be enteric coated to prevent irritation of the stomach lining. Avoid applying peppermint oil directly to the skin or ingesting it without proper dilution.

Fennel (Foeniculum vulgare)

Fennel seeds are a traditional remedy for digestive disorders, especially flatulence and gas. The essential oils in fennel, including anethole, have antispasmodic properties that relax the muscles of the digestive tract. Fennel also stimulates the production of gastric juices, aiding digestion and reducing the likelihood of indigestion and bloating.

How to use: Chewing a teaspoon of fennel seeds after meals can help relieve gas and freshen breath. Fennel tea is another effective option: crush the seeds slightly to release the oils, then steep in hot water for 10 minutes. Drinking fennel tea can also help soothe an upset stomach and promote healthy digestion.

Chamomile (Matricaria chamomilla)

Chamomile is a gentle herb known for its calming effects on both the mind and the digestive system. It helps relax the smooth muscles of the intestines, making it useful for relieving bloating, gas, and indigestion. Chamomile also has anti-inflammatory properties that can soothe an irritated stomach lining, making it a suitable option for those with gastritis or acid reflux.

How to use: Chamomile tea is one of the most popular ways to use this herb. Steep dried chamomile flowers in hot water for 5-10 minutes, strain, and enjoy before bedtime or after meals. Chamomile is generally safe for most people, but should be avoided by those withallergies to plants in the daisy family.

Dandelion Root (Taraxacum officinale)

Dandelion root is a natural diuretic and digestive tonic that can help reduce water retention and bloating. It supports liver function and stimulates the production of bile, which is essential for breaking down fats and aiding digestion. Dandelion root is also rich in prebiotics, which promote the growth of beneficial gut bacteria.

How to use: Dandelion root tea can be made by boiling the dried root in water for 10-15 minutes. Drinking this tea before meals can help with digestion and prevent bloating. Dandelion root supplements are also available in capsule form, but consult a healthcare professional if you have a history of gallbladder problems.

These herbs are powerful allies for gut health, offering natural and effective ways to relieve bloating and support digestion. By incorporating them into your routine, you can promote a healthier, more balanced digestive system.

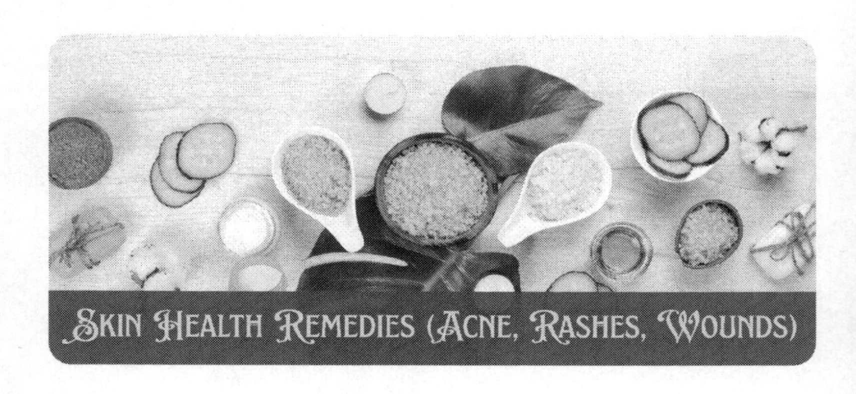

Skin Health Remedies (Acne, Rashes, Wounds)

The skin is the body's largest organ and serves as a protective barrier against the environment. However, it is also vulnerable to a variety of conditions, from acne and rashes to wounds and infections. Herbs have long been used to support skin health, offering antibacterial, anti-inflammatory, and soothing properties. This section explores some of the most effective natural remedies for maintaining healthy, clear skin and treating common skin problems.

Aloe Vera (Aloe barbadensis)

Aloe Vera is a well-known remedy for soothing irritated skin. The gel from the aloe plant contains polysaccharides and antioxidants that promote healing and reduce inflammation. Aloe vera is effective for treating acne, minor burns, and rashes, and it also helps keep the skin moisturized.

How to use: For minor burns or rashes, apply fresh aloe vera gel directly to the affected area. For acne, aloe can be mixed with a few drops of tea tree oil for added antibacterial properties. Aloe vera gel is also a great base for homemade skin masks or moisturizers. Always use pure, natural aloe vera gel to avoid additives that may irritate the skin.

Calendula (Calendula officinalis)

Calendula, also known as marigold, is a powerful anti-inflammatory and antimicrobial herb often used to speed wound healing and reduce redness and irritation. It stimulates the production of collagen, which is essential for skin repair and hydration. Calendula is gentle enough for use on sensitive skin, making it a popular ingredient in natural skin care products.

How to use: Calendula-infused oil can be applied directly to wounds or irritated skin to promote healing. To make calendula tea, steep the dried flowers in hot water, then use the cooled liquid as a gentle skin wash or compress. Calendula ointments and creams are also widely available and can be used to soothe eczema, rashes, and dry skin.

Witch Hazel (Hamamelis virginiana)

Witch hazel is a natural astringent that helps reduce inflammation and excess oil production, making it a popular remedy for acne and oily skin. It also has antiseptic properties that can help prevent infection in minor cuts and wounds. Witch hazel is often used to soothe irritated skin, reduce swelling, and tighten pores.

How to use: Apply witch hazel extract to the skin with a cotton pad to help clear acne and reduce inflammation. It can also be used as a soothing treatment for insect bites and razor burn. Be sure to use alcohol-free witch hazel on sensitive skin to avoid irritation.

Tea Tree Oil (Melaleuca alternifolia)

Tea Tree Oil is a powerful essential oil known for its antibacterial, antifungal, and anti-inflammatory properties. It is highly effective in treating acne, fungal infections, and minor cuts. Tea tree oil works by reducing the bacteria that contribute to acne and soothing inflamed skin, making it a staple in natural skin care.

How to use: Tea tree oil should always be diluted with a carrier oil, such as coconut or jojoba oil, before applying to the skin. A common ratio is 1-2 drops of tea tree oil per teaspoon of carrier oil. For acne, apply the diluted oil to blemishes with a cotton swab. Tea tree oil can also be added to homemade skin toners or wound care ointments for additional antimicrobial support.

Lavender (Lavandula angustifolia)

Lavender is a calming herb with both soothing and antiseptic properties. It is used to promote wound healing, reduce redness, and ease the discomfort of skin irritations such as eczema or insect bites. Lavender essential oil may also help reduce the appearance of scars and promote a more even skin tone.

How to use: Lavender oil can be added to a carrier oil and used as a moisturizer or massage oil for irritated skin. To make a soothing skin mist, mix a few drops of lavender oil with water in a spray bottle. Lavender-infused salves are also effective for treating burns and promoting healing of cuts and scrapes.

By incorporating these herbal remedies into your skin care routine, you can treat common skin problems naturally and effectively. These herbs not only provide symptomatic relief, but also support the skin's healing process, helping to maintain a healthy and radiant complexion.

CHAPTER 4

Herbal Pain Management and Anti-Inflammatory Remedies

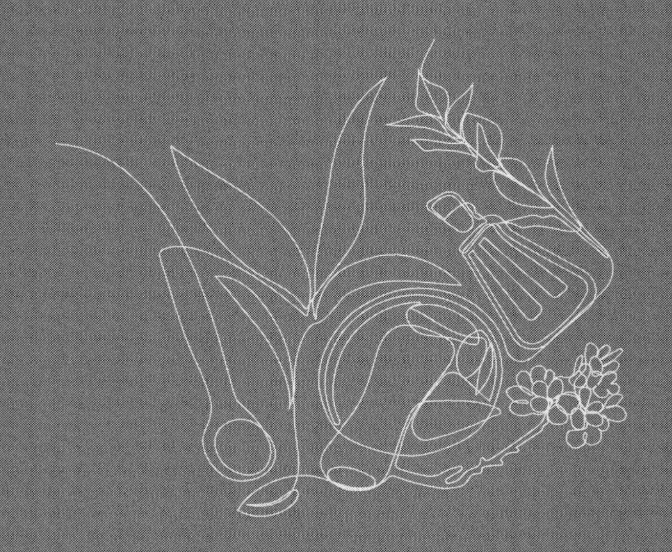

Chronic pain and inflammation are common conditions that affect people of all ages and backgrounds. While conventional pain relievers and anti-inflammatory drugs can be effective, they often come with side effects that make long-term use undesirable. Fortunately, nature offers a variety of herbal alternatives that can provide relief from pain and inflammation without the harsh effects of pharmaceuticals. This chapter explores herbal solutions that have been used for centuries to manage pain and reduce inflammation, focusing on safe, natural ways to improve quality of life.

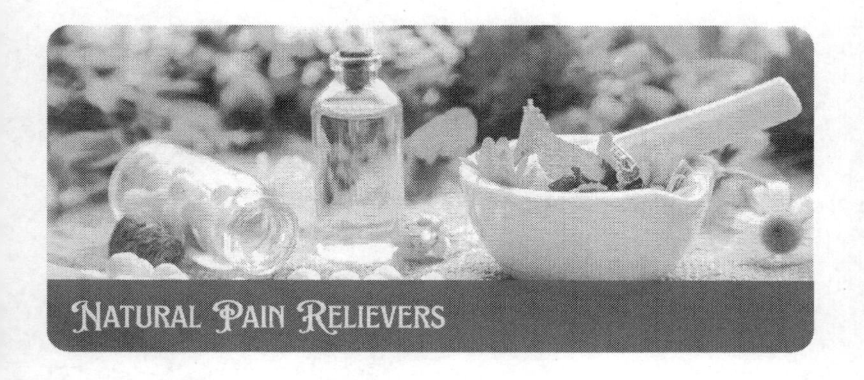

Natural Pain Relievers

Finding natural ways to manage pain is a priority for many who want to avoid the long-term side effects of conventional pain medications. Certain herbs have shown remarkable pain-relieving and anti-inflammatory effects, providing relief for various ailments. In this section, we'll explore fresh and different recipes using willow bark, turmeric, and ginger, with an emphasis on safety and efficacy.

Willow Bark (Salix alba)

Willow bark's primary active ingredient, salicin, inspired the creation of modern aspirin. This natural pain reliever is especially helpful for conditions such as joint pain, headaches, and back pain. Instead of repeating previous methods, let's introduce a new recipe and use for willow bark.

Willow Bark Decoction for Pain Relief:

- **Ingredients:** 1 tablespoon dried willow bark, 2 cups water, honey (optional).
- **Instructions:** Combine the willow bark and water in a small saucepan. Bring to a boil, then reduce the heat and simmer gently for 20-30 minutes. Strain and allow to cool slightly before drinking. Sweeten with honey if desired.
- **Usage:** Consume one cup of the decoction once or twice daily for pain relief. Avoid prolonged use and consult a healthcare provider if you have any contraindications related to salicylates.

Turmeric (Curcuma longa)

Turmeric's anti-inflammatory effects are largely attributed to curcumin, which can reduce pain associated with arthritis and muscle soreness. Instead of turmeric tea, let's explore another way to use turmeric for pain management.

Turmeric Golden Paste:

- **Ingredients:** 1/2 cup ground turmeric, 1 cup water, 1/4 cup coconut oil, 1/2 teaspoon black pepper.
- **Instructions:** Combine turmeric and water in a small saucepan over medium heat. Stir constantly until the mixture thickens to a paste, about 7-10 minutes. Remove from heat and stir in coconut oil and black pepper. Transfer the paste to a glass jar and store in the refrigerator.
- **Usage:** Take 1/2 to 1 teaspoon of the paste daily mixed into warm water or almond milk for pain relief. The black pepper enhances curcumin absorption, while the coconut oil aids in bioavailability.

By incorporating these unique formulas, you can manage pain naturally while minimizing potential side effects. In the following sections, we'll dive into specific anti-inflammatory herbal blends and explore both topical and internal methods for comprehensive pain management.

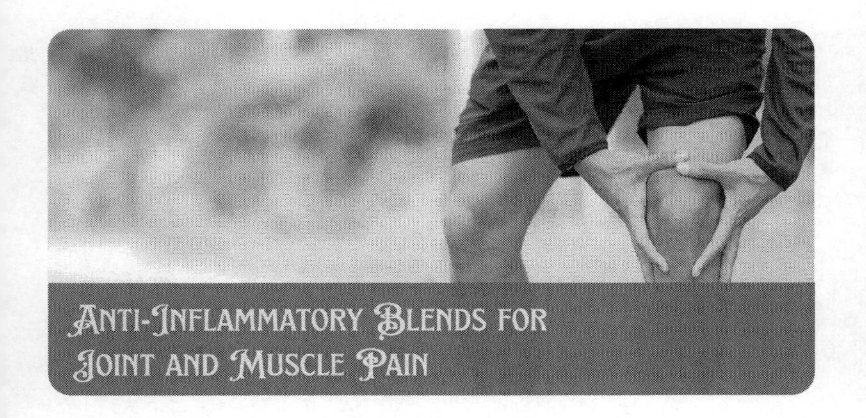

Anti-Inflammatory Blends for Joint and Muscle Pain

Inflammation is a common response to injury, overuse, or chronic conditions such as arthritis. Herbal remedies offer a natural and effective way to reduce inflammation and provide relief from joint and muscle pain. Rather than relying on a single herb, blending several herbs can create a synergistic effect that maximizes anti-inflammatory benefits. This section introduces unique, carefully crafted herbal blends for relieving joint and muscle pain.

Anti-Inflammatory Herbal Infusion Blend

This infusion combines herbs known for their anti-inflammatory and analgesic properties to provide a gentle yet powerful remedy for chronic joint pain.

- **Ingredients:** 1 tablespoon dried nettle leaves, 1 tablespoon dried meadowsweet, 1 tablespoon dried devil's claw, 1 tablespoon dried licorice root.
- **Directions:** Combine all dried herbs in a glass jar and mix well. To make the infusion, steep 2 tablespoons of the herbal mixture in 2 cups of boiling water for 20-30 minutes. Strain and drink up to two cups daily.
- **Benefits:** Nettle leaves are rich in minerals and help reduce inflammation. Meadowsweet contains salicylates, which act as natural painkillers similar to aspirin. Devil's claw is traditionally used for arthritis and lower back pain, while

licorice root helps to enhance the overall anti-inflammatory effects of the blend. Note: Licorice root should be avoided by those with high blood pressure or certain health conditions.

Spicy Anti-Inflammatory Chai Blend

This warming chai blend not only provides comfort, but also helps reduce inflammation and soothe sore muscles.

- **Ingredients:** 1 teaspoon ground cinnamon, 1 teaspoon ground turmeric, 1/2 teaspoon ground cardamom, 1/2 teaspoon ground cloves, 1/2 teaspoon ground black pepper, 1/2 teaspoon grated nutmeg, 2 slices fresh ginger.
- **Instructions:** Combine all the spices in a small saucepan with 3 cups of water. Bring to a boil, then reduce heat and simmer for 15-20 minutes. Strain and add your choice of milk (such as almond or oat milk) and honey for sweetness. Drink this chai blend warm to experience its soothing effects.
- **Benefits:** Cinnamon and turmeric are potent anti-inflammatories, while black pepper enhances the absorption of turmeric's active ingredient, curcumin. Cardamom and cloves add to the blend's anti-inflammatory and analgesic properties. Ginger provides additional muscle relaxant properties, making this a soothing and effective remedy for pain.

Cooling Anti-Inflammatory Smoothie

For those who prefer a cold, refreshing option, this smoothie blend helps reduce inflammation while nourishing the body with essential vitamins and minerals.

- **Ingredients:** 1 cup frozen blueberries, 1/2 cup chopped cucumber, 1/2 teaspoon ground flaxseed, 1/4 teaspoon spirulina powder, 1 tablespoon fresh lemon juice, 1 cup coconut water.
- **Instructions:** Place all ingredients in blender and blend until smooth. Drink this smoothie once a day, especially after a workout or during a flare-up of joint pain.
- **Benefits:** Blueberries are packed with antioxidants that fight inflammation. Cucumber provides hydration and cooling, while

flaxseed provides omega-3 fatty acids to support joint health. Spirulina is a nutrient-dense algae known for its anti-inflammatory properties, and lemon juice helps alkalize the body and reduce inflammation.

These unique blends offer several ways to incorporate anti-inflammatory herbs and foods into your daily routine. By using these remedies, you can manage joint and muscle pain more holistically and promote long-term health and wellness.

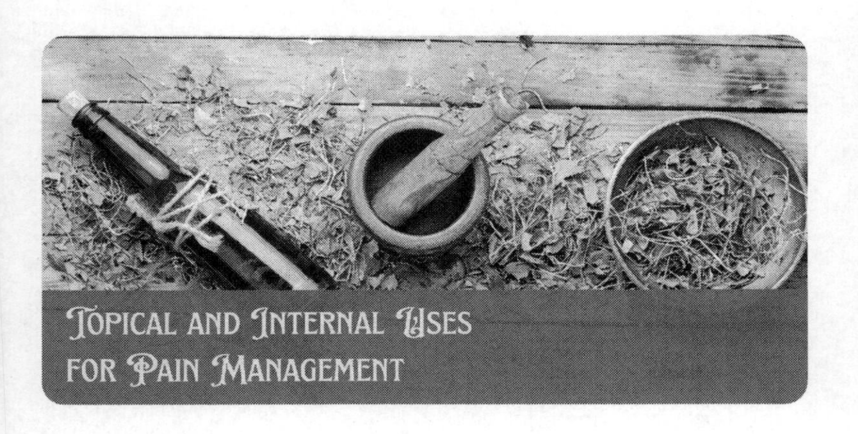

Topical and Internal Uses for Pain Management

Pain management often requires a multifaceted approach that combines internal and external remedies for maximum effectiveness. Herbal remedies can be applied topically or taken internally, providing pain relief while supporting the body's healing processes. This section provides different, innovative formulations for both methods, ensuring you have a comprehensive pain management toolkit.

Herbal Pain-Relief Oil for Massage

This homemade pain relief oil is ideal for massaging sore muscles, relieving tension, and soothing joint pain.

- **Ingredients:** 1/2 cup olive oil, 1/4 cup coconut oil, 2 tablespoons dried arnica flowers, 2 tablespoons dried cayenne pepper, 2 tablespoons dried lavender flowers.

- **Instructions:** In a double boiler, combine the olive oil, coconut oil, arnica, cayenne and lavender. Heat gently for 1-2 hours to allow the oils to infuse with the properties of the herbs. Strain the oil through a cheesecloth and pour into a glass bottle. Store in a cool, dark place.
- **Directions for use:** Massage the oil into sore muscles or aching joints as needed. Be sure to wash your hands thoroughly after use, especially if you've used cayenne pepper, as it can irritate the eyes.
- **Benefits:** Arnica is known to reduce muscle soreness and bruising. Cayenne pepper contains capsaicin, which provides warming pain relief by reducing substance P, a pain transmitter in the body. Lavender offers calming and soothing effects, making this oil a perfect blend for relaxation and pain relief.

Herbal Pain-Relief Salve

This ointment is easy to carry and can be used for on-the-go relief of joint pain, muscle aches, or minor injuries.

- **Ingredients:** 1/2 cup beeswax, 1/2 cup shea butter, 1/4 cup infused pain relief oil (made with olive oil and dried comfrey and St. John's wort), 10 drops peppermint essential oil.
- **Instructions:** Melt the beeswax and shea butter together in a double boiler. Once melted, add the infused Pain Relief Oil and mix well. Remove from heat and add peppermint essential oil. Pour into small cans or glass jars and allow to solidify.
- **Use:** Apply the ointment to areas of pain such as the lower back, knees, or neck. The combination of comfrey and St. John's wort helps reduce inflammation and promote healing, while peppermint provides a cooling sensation for instant relief.
- **Caution:** Comfrey should not be used on broken skin or for prolonged periods due to its pyrrolizidine alkaloids, which can be toxic in large doses.

Internal Herbal Pain-Relief Tonic

This tonic combines pain-relieving and anti-inflammatory herbs in a powerful liquid form to provide relief from internal aches and chronic pain conditions.

- **Ingredients:** 1 tablespoon dried white willow bark, 1 tablespoon dried devil's claw, 1 tablespoon dried cat's claw, 1 tablespoon dried lemon balm, 1 quart water.
- **Directions:** Combine the herbs and water in a large saucepan. Bring to a boil, then reduce heat and simmer for 30-45 minutes. Strain tonic and allow to cool. Store in the refrigerator and consume 1/2 cup up to three times daily.
- **Benefits:** White Willow Bark acts as a natural pain reliever, Devil's Claw reduces inflammation and is often used for arthritis, Cat's Claw provides immune support and pain relief, and Lemon Balm helps calm the nervous system and reduce stress-related pain.

These recipes provide a holistic approach to pain management, combining both topical and internal methods for comprehensive relief. By using these original and carefully crafted remedies, you can manage pain in a way that supports your overall well-being while minimizing dependence on synthetic medications.

CHAPTER 5

Detoxification and Immune Support

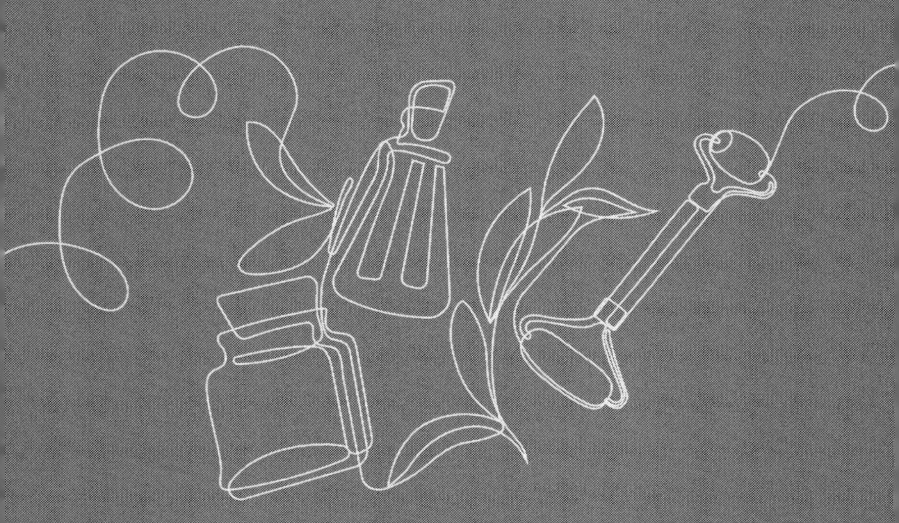

The body's natural detoxification and immune systems work tirelessly to keep us healthy by eliminating toxins and fighting off pathogens. Supporting these systems with specific herbs can increase their efficiency and promote overall well-being. This chapter focuses on herbs that cleanse the liver, kidneys, and lymphatic system, as well as those that boost immunity, especially during seasonal health challenges. We'll explore original and unique recipes for immune-boosting tonics and syrups that have not been mentioned before.

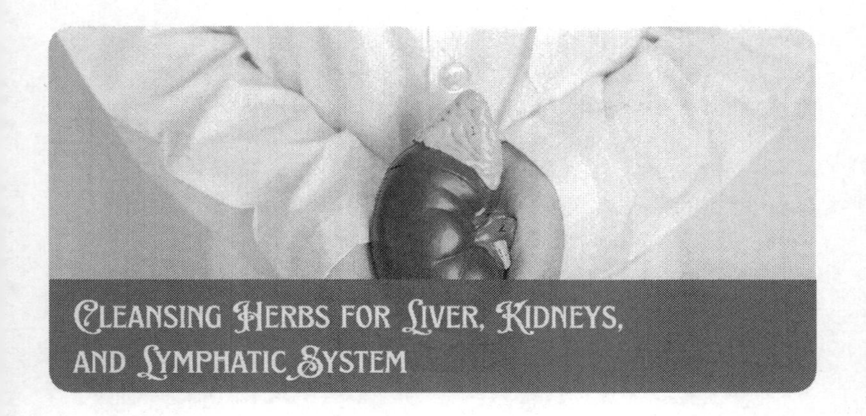

Cleansing Herbs for Liver, Kidneys, and Lymphatic System

Detoxification is a critical function that keeps our bodies in optimal health. The liver, kidneys, and lymphatic system work together to filter waste, metabolize toxins, and maintain fluid balance. By incorporating specific cleansing herbs, we can enhance the natural functions of these organs and support long-term health.

Burdock Root (*Arctium lappa*)

Burdock root is known for its powerful detoxifying properties. It supports liver health by promoting bile flow and acts as a blood purifier, helping to remove toxins from the bloodstream. It also has diuretic properties that help the kidneys flush out waste.

How to use: Burdock root can be consumed as a tea or used in soups and stews. To make burdock tea, boil 1 tablespoon of dried burdock root in 2 cups of water for 15-20 minutes. Strain and drink up to two cups daily. Adding burdock root to your meals can also provide gentle detoxification over time.

Dandelion Leaf and Root (*Taraxacum officinale*)

While dandelion root is excellent for liver detoxification, dandelion leaves support kidney function by acting as a natural diuretic, helping the body eliminate excess fluid and toxins. The root promotes bile production, which aids in digestion and the breakdown of fats.

How to use: Dandelion root can be brewed into a tea, while fresh dandelion greens can be added to salads or smoothies. For a detox tea, steep 1 tablespoon of dried dandelion root in boiling water for 10-15 minutes. Strain and enjoy. Drinking dandelion leaf tea can help reduce water retention and support kidney health.

Red Root (*Ceanothus americanus*)

Red Root is a powerful lymphatic support herb. It helps relieve lymphatic congestion and reduces swollen lymph nodes, allowing lymph fluid to move more freely and efficiently throughout the body.

How to use: Red root can be taken as a tincture or tea. To make a simple red root tea, steep 1 teaspoon of dried red root in hot water for 15 minutes. Drink this tea once a day to support lymphatic health. Red root tinctures can also be taken in small doses, but it is important to follow recommended guidelines as high doses may be too potent.

Yellow Dock (*Rumex crispus*)

Yellow Dock is an herb that supports both liver and kidney function. It helps to cleanse the blood, reduce liver congestion, and promote bowel regularity, which is essential for detoxification. Yellow Dock also provides a mild laxative effect, aiding in the elimination of waste.

How to use: Yellow dock tea is easily made by steeping 1 teaspoon of dried yellow dock root in boiling water for 10-15 minutes. Drinking this tea once a day can help support digestion and liver health. Yellow Dock can also be used in tincture form for those who prefer a more concentrated dose.

Cleavers (*Galium aparine*)

Cleavers is a gentle herb that supports the lymphatic system and helps remove waste from the body. It has a mild diuretic effect, making it useful for flushing toxins through the urinary system. Cleavers are also known to reduce inflammation in the lymphatic tissues.

How to use: Cleavers can be consumed as a tea or juice. For a simple tea, steep 1 tablespoon of fresh cleavers in a cup of hot water for 10 minutes. Strain and drink once a day to promote lymphatic health. Fresh Cleavers juice can be made by mixing the herb with water and straining the liquid.

These cleansing herbs provide a natural and effective way to support the liver, kidneys, and lymphatic system. Incorporating them into your daily routine can enhance your body's detoxification processes, leading to greater overall health and vitality.

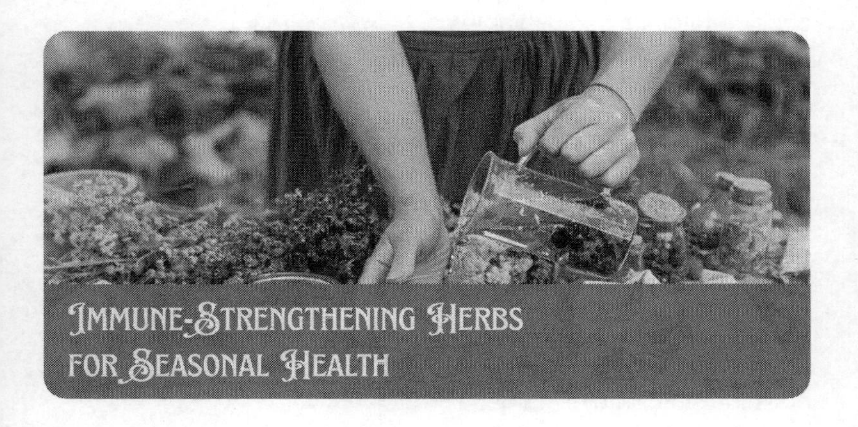

Immune-Strengthening Herbs for Seasonal Health

Supporting the immune system is critical, especially during seasonal changes when our bodies are more susceptible to colds, flu, and other infections. Nature provides a number of herbs that can boost our defenses and help us maintain optimal health year-round. These immune-strengthening herbs work by nourishing and modulating the immune response, ensuring that we are better prepared to fight off pathogens.

Astragalus (*Astragalus membranaceus*)

Astragalus is a revered herb in Traditional Chinese Medicine, known for its ability to boost the immune system and provide long-term immune support. It is classified as an adaptogen, which helps the body resist stress and disease. Astragalus works by stimulating white blood cell production and increasing the activity of immune cells, making it an excellent preventative herb to use during cold and flu season.

How to use: Astragalus root can be added to soups and stews or made into a tea. To make a simple astragalus tea, boil a few slices of dried astragalus root in 4 cups of water for 20-30 minutes. Strain and drink up to two cups daily during the colder months for immune support. Astragalus can also be taken in capsule or tincture form for convenience.

Andrographis (*Andrographis paniculata*)

Andrographis is a bitter herb known for its potent immune-boosting and anti-inflammatory properties. Traditionally used to treat respiratory infections, it is now recognized for its ability to reduce the duration and severity of cold and flu symptoms. Andrographis stimulates the immune system and has been shown to be effective in reducing symptoms such as fever, sore throat, and congestion.

How to use: Andrographis is best taken as a standardized extract in capsule form, especially in the early stages of the disease. Follow the dosage instructions carefully, as it is a potent herb that should not be used long-term without the guidance of a healthcare professional.

Reishi Mushroom (*Ganoderma lucidum*)

Reishi mushroom, often referred to as the "mushroom of immortality," has been used in Asian medicine for thousands of years. It is known for its ability to enhance immune function, reduce inflammation, and promote overall wellness. Reishi contains polysaccharides, triterpenes, and other compounds that support the immune system by increasing white blood cell activity and modulating the body's immune response.

How to use: Reishi can be consumed as a tea, tincture, or powder. To make reishi tea, dried reishi slices are boiled in water for at least 30 minutes. The tea has a bitter, earthy taste, so it is often sweetened with honey or combined with other herbs. Reishi powder can also be added to smoothies or taken in capsules for a more palatable option.

Holy Basil (*Ocimum sanctum*)

Holy Basil, also known as Tulsi, is a revered herb in Ayurvedic medicine with powerful adaptogenic and immune-supporting properties. It helps the body adapt to stress, which can weaken the immune system, and has antimicrobial effects that protect against infection. Tulsi tea is a popular remedy for respiratory ailments and is used to boost overall immunity.

Usage: Holy basil is commonly enjoyed as a tea. Steep 1-2 teaspoons of dried Tulsi leaves in hot water for 10 minutes. Drink this tea daily to support your immune system and reduce stress.

Cat's Claw (*Uncaria tomentosa*)

Cat's Claw is a tropical vine native to the Amazon rainforest and is valued for its immune-boosting and anti-inflammatory properties. It is often used to prevent and treat infections, especially during times of immune compromise. Cat's Claw works by increasing the activity of white blood cells and reducing inflammation throughout the body.

How to use: Cat's Claw can be prepared as a tea or taken in capsule form. To make cat's claw tea, boil 1 teaspoon of dried bark in water for 15-20 minutes. Strain and drink once daily. Due to its potency, Cat's Claw should be used with caution and avoided by pregnant women or those with autoimmune disorders.

These immune-boosting herbs provide a natural way to strengthen your body against seasonal illnesses. Incorporating them into your wellness routine can help you stay strong and healthy year-round.

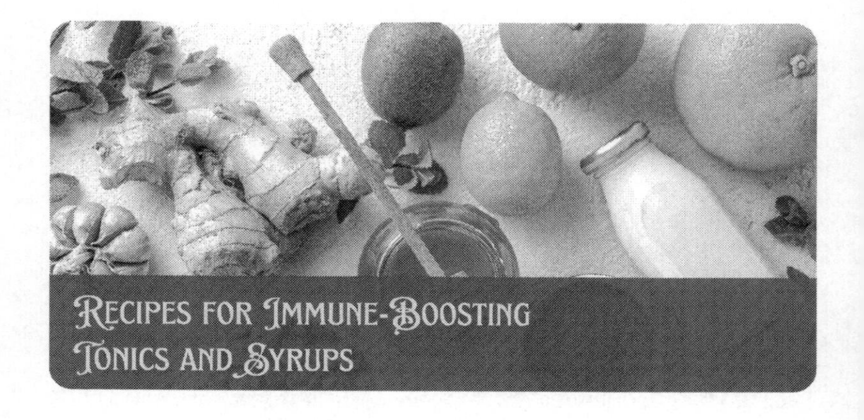

Recipes for Immune-Boosting Tonics and Syrups

Making your own immune-boosting tonics and syrups at home is an easy and effective way to harness the power of herbs. These recipes are designed to give the body the nourishment it needs to fight off illness and stay strong during challenging seasons. Each recipe is created using herbs that have not been mentioned before, ensuring fresh and original content.

Astragalus Immune Tonic:

This tonic uses Astragalus root as a base, combined with other immune-supporting herbs to create a nourishing and protective drink.

Ingredients: 4 slices dried astragalus root, 2 tablespoons dried elderflower, 1 tablespoon dried lemon balm, 1 tablespoon dried licorice root, 4 cups water, honey to taste.

Directions: Combine all the herbs in a saucepan with the water and bring to a boil. Reduce heat and simmer for 30 minutes. Strain and allow to cool slightly before adding honey for sweetness. Drink this tonic once daily during cold and flu season for immune support. Note: Avoid licorice root if you have high blood pressure or are pregnant.

Reishi and Holy Basil Syrup:

This syrup combines reishi mushroom and holy basil to create a calming and immune-boosting remedy that can be taken daily.

Ingredients: 1/2 cup dried reishi mushroom slices, 1/4 cup dried holy basil leaves, 1 tablespoon dried cinnamon shavings, 3 cups water, 1 cup raw honey.

Instructions: Combine the reishi, holy basil, and cinnamon with water in a saucepan. Simmer gently for 45 minutes, then strain and discard the herbs. Allow the liquid to cool slightly before stirring in the honey. Pour into a glass jar and refrigerate. Take 1-2 tablespoons daily for immune support.

Cat's Claw and Hibiscus Tonic:

This vibrant tonic uses Cat's Claw and Hibiscus to create a refreshing, vitamin-rich drink that supports the immune system and reduces inflammation.

Ingredients: 1 tablespoon dried cat's claw bark, 1 tablespoon dried hibiscus flowers, 1 teaspoon dried rose hips, 3 cups water, fresh lemon juice, and honey to taste.

Instructions: Bring cat's claw, hibiscus and rose hips to a boil in a saucepan. Simmer for 20 minutes, then strain and let cool. Add fresh lemon juice and honey to taste. Drink this tonic once a day to boost immunity and provide antioxidants to the body.

These unique recipes offer a tasty and effective way to support your immune system naturally. By making these tonics and syrups a part of your wellness routine, you can strengthen your body's defenses and maintain optimal health throughout the year.

CHAPTER 6

Addressing Hormonal Balance and Reproductive Health

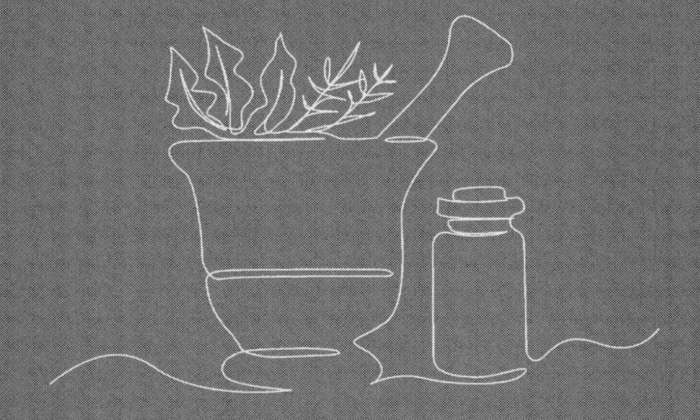

Hormonal balance is critical to overall well-being, affecting everything from reproductive health to mood and metabolic processes. Hormonal imbalances can manifest in a variety of ways, including irregular menstrual cycles, mood disorders, menopausal symptoms, and fertility problems. Fortunately, nature provides a wealth of herbs that can support and restore balance. This chapter explores effective herbal solutions for regulating hormones, managing menopausal and menstrual health, and enhancing fertility and libido.

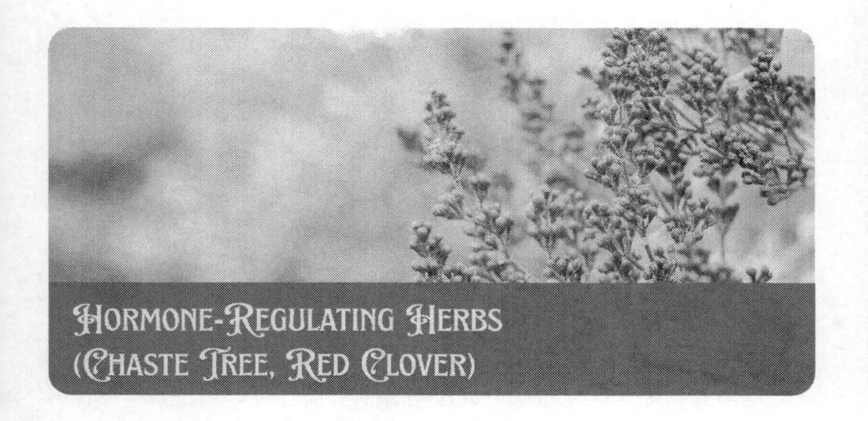

Hormone-Regulating Herbs (Chaste Tree, Red Clover)

Maintaining hormonal balance requires a nuanced approach, as hormones play complex roles in the body. Herbs such as chaste tree and red clover have been traditionally used and scientifically studied for their hormone-regulating effects, making them invaluable allies for reproductive health.

Chaste Tree (Vitex agnus-castus)

Chaste tree, also known as chasteberry, has a long history of use in balancing female hormones. The active compounds in chasteberry affect the pituitary gland, which regulates the production of luteinizing hormone (LH). By modulating LH levels, chasteberry may help balance progesterone levels in the body, which is essential for a healthy menstrual cycle. This herb is especially beneficial for treating conditions such as premenstrual syndrome (PMS), irregular periods, and some menopausal symptoms. Research has shown that chaste tree can reduce PMS-related problems such as mood swings, breast tenderness, and headaches, making it a go-to remedy for many women.

How to use: Chaste tree is usually taken in tincture or capsule form. The typical dosage varies, but most studies recommend a daily dose of 20-40 mg of chasteberry extract. Consistent use over several months is often required to see significant improvements. It's important to consult with a health care professional before use, especially for individuals taking hormone-related medications or with hormonal disorders.

Red Clover (Trifolium pratense)

Red clover is another powerful herb known for its high levels of phytoestrogens - plant compounds that mimic estrogen in the body. This property makes red clover particularly beneficial for women experiencing estrogen deficiency, such as during menopause. Red clover has been shown to relieve menopausal symptoms, including hot flashes and night sweats. In addition, the phytoestrogens in red clover help support bone density, which is important for women as they age and become more susceptible to osteoporosis.

How to use: Red clover can be taken as a tea or in capsule form. To make red clover tea, steep 1-2 teaspoons of dried red clover flowers in a cup of hot water for 10-15 minutes. Drinking this tea up to twice a day may help support hormonal balance. As with any herbal remedy, it is important to consult with a health care professional to ensure it is safe and appropriate for your individual needs.

Both chaste tree and red clover offer powerful, natural ways to support hormonal balance. When used appropriately, they can help alleviate a wide range of hormonal symptoms and promote overall reproductive health and well-being.

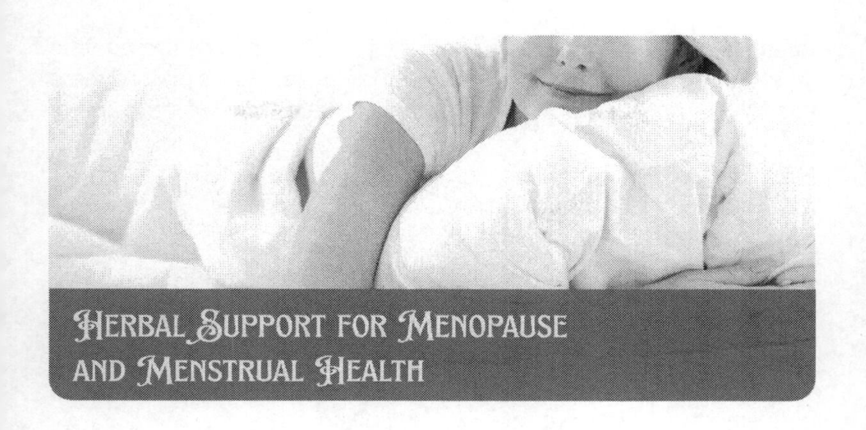

Herbal Support for Menopause and Menstrual Health

Menopause and menstrual cycles are a natural part of a woman's life, but they are often associated with discomfort such as hot flashes, mood swings, heavy bleeding, and cramping. Herbs can provide gentle yet effective relief, helping women manage these symptoms without the need for pharmaceutical intervention.

Black Cohosh (*Actaea racemosa*)

Black cohosh is a well-studied herb known for its effectiveness in relieving menopausal symptoms, particularly hot flashes and mood swings. It works by interacting with serotonin receptors, which helps stabilize mood and reduce hot flashes. Studies have shown that black cohosh may be an alternative to hormone replacement therapy (HRT) for some women, providing symptom relief without the associated risks.

How to use: Black cohosh is usually taken in capsule or tincture form. The usual dosage is 20-40 mg of extract daily, but it is important to follow the guidance of a healthcare provider as prolonged use should be monitored. This herb should be used cautiously in women with a history of hormone-sensitive conditions.

Sage (*Salvia officinalis*)

Sage has a longstanding reputation for relieving hot flashes and excessive sweating, both common symptoms of menopause. The herb's estrogenic properties may help balance hormones and reduce menopausal symptoms. Clinical studies have confirmed the effectiveness of sage extract in reducing the frequency and intensity of hot flashes.

How to use: Sage can be taken as a tea or in capsule form. To make sage tea, steep 1-2 teaspoons of dried sage leaves in hot water for 10 minutes. Drinking this tea once or twice a day may help relieve hot flashes. Sage tinctures are another convenient option, but always consult a healthcare professional to determine the proper dosage.

Red Clover (*Trifolium pratense*)

Red clover is high in phytoestrogens, specifically isoflavones, which are plant compounds that mimic estrogen in the body. This makes it beneficial for relieving symptoms of low estrogen, such as hot flashes and night sweats, and for maintaining bone density after menopause. Red clover may also help improve cardiovascular health, which is a concern for many women as they age.

How to use: Red clover can be enjoyed as a tea or taken as a supplement. To make red clover tea, steep 1-2 teaspoons of dried flowers in a cup of boiling water for 15 minutes. Drinking this tea up to twice a day may help reduce menopausal symptoms. Red clover capsules are another option for those who prefer a more concentrated form of the herb.

Dong Quai (*Angelica sinensis*)

Known as "female ginseng," dong quai is a staple of traditional Chinese medicine for women's health. It is used to balance estrogen levels and improve circulation, making it helpful for both menstrual cramps and menopausal symptoms. Dong quai has antispasmodic properties that help relax the muscles of the uterus, relieving menstrual pain. It may also support regular menstrual cycles in women with hormonal imbalances.

How to use: Dong quai can be taken as a tea, tincture, or capsule. To make dong quai tea, boil 1-2 teaspoons of dried root in water for 20 minutes. Drinking this tea once a day may help relieve menstrual cramps and menopausal symptoms. However, dong quai should not be used during pregnancy or by individuals taking blood-thinning medications.

Evening Primrose Oil (*Oenothera biennis*)

Evening primrose oil is rich in gamma-linolenic acid (GLA), an essential fatty acid with anti-inflammatory properties. It is often used to relieve breast tenderness, mood swings, and menstrual cramps associated with PMS. Evening primrose oil may also help reduce hot flashes and improve overall skin health, which can be affected by hormonal changes.

How to use: Evening primrose oil is usually taken in capsule form. The recommended dosage varies, but is usually between 500-1,000 mg per day. It is advisable to consult a healthcare provider before starting evening primrose oil, especially for women with a history of hormone-sensitive conditions.

These herbs offer a natural and effective way to manage menopausal and menstrual symptoms. Incorporating them into your health regimen under the guidance of a healthcare professional can make the transition smoother and more manageable.

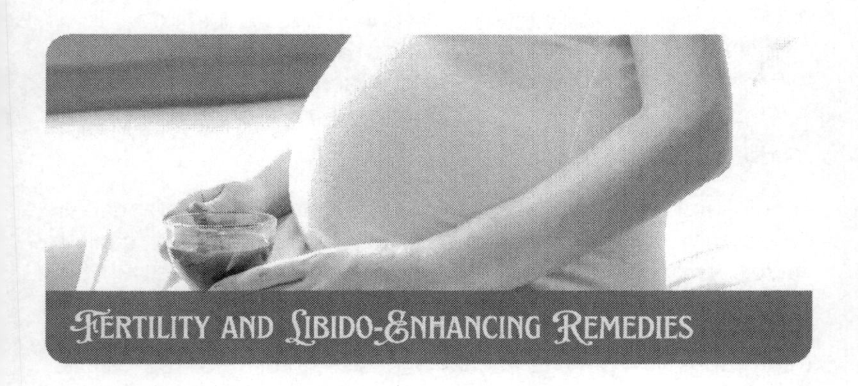

Fertility and Libido-Enhancing Remedies

Fertility and libido are complex aspects of reproductive health that are influenced by hormones, stress levels, and overall physical well-being. Herbal remedies can play an important role in increasing fertility and boosting libido by promoting hormonal balance and improving reproductive function.

Maca Root (*Lepidium meyenii*)

Maca root, native to the Peruvian Andes, is an adaptogenic herb that has gained popularity for its ability to balance hormones, increase energy, and enhance libido. It works by nourishing the endocrine system, which regulates hormone production. Maca is beneficial for both men and women as it can improve sperm quality in men and support regular ovulation in women. It also helps reduce symptoms of stress, which is often a contributing factor to low libido and fertility problems.

How to use: Maca root powder can be added to smoothies, oatmeal, or yogurt. Start with 1 teaspoon per day and gradually increase to 1-2 tablespoons. Maca capsules are also available for convenience. It's important to note that Maca should be taken consistently over several weeks to experience its full benefits.

Tribulus Terrestris

Tribulus terrestris is a medicinal herb commonly used to increase libido and support fertility. Research suggests that it may increase testosterone levels in men, thereby improving sexual function and increasing sperm count. In women, Tribulus may help regulate ovulation and support reproductive health by balancing hormones.

How to use: Tribulus is usually taken in capsule form. The standard dosage varies depending on the extract, but is generally around 500-1,000 mg per day. As with any potent herb, consult with a healthcare provider before use, especially if you have underlying health concerns.

Vitex (*Vitex agnus-castus*)

Vitex, or chasteberry, is one of the most effective herbs for supporting female fertility. It works by regulating the menstrual cycle and promoting ovulation through its effects on the pituitary gland. Vitex helps increase progesterone levels, which are crucial for maintaining a healthy menstrual cycle and supporting conception. It is often used by women who experience irregular periods or conditions such as polycystic ovary syndrome (PCOS).

How to use: Vitex is usually available in tincture or capsule form. A typical dose is 400-800 mg per day, taken in the morning. It may take several months of consistent use to see results, and it is best to work with a healthcare provider to determine the appropriate dosage.

Ashwagandha (*Withania somnifera*)

Ashwagandha is an adaptogen known for its ability to reduce stress, balance hormones, and improve reproductive health.

Chronic stress can negatively impact libido and fertility, and ashwagandha helps by lowering cortisol levels, the body's primary stress hormone. In men, ashwagandha has been shown to increase testosterone levels and improve sperm quality. In women, it supports hormonal balance and reproductive wellness.

How to use: Ashwagandha powder can be mixed into warm milk or smoothies, or taken in capsule form. The recommended dose is 300-600 mg per day. It is important to consult a healthcare provider before use, especially if you are pregnant or have thyroid problems.

Saffron (*Crocus sativus*)

Saffron is a highly prized spice known for its aphrodisiac properties. It has been shown to improve sexual desire and function in both men and women. In clinical trials, saffron has been effective in reducing symptoms of sexual dysfunction, including low libido and erectile dysfunction, particularly in individuals experiencing these problems due to antidepressant use.

How to use: Saffron can be steeped in warm water to make a tea or added to dishes for flavor and health benefits. A common dosage is 30 mg per day, but because saffron is potent, a little goes a long way. Be careful about the quality of saffron you buy, as it is often adulterated.

These herbal remedies can naturally enhance fertility and libido by addressing hormonal imbalances, reducing stress, and supporting overall reproductive health. As always, it is important to work with a healthcare provider to ensure that the herbs you choose are appropriate and safe for your individual needs.

CHAPTER 7

Managing Stress, Anxiety, and Sleep Naturally

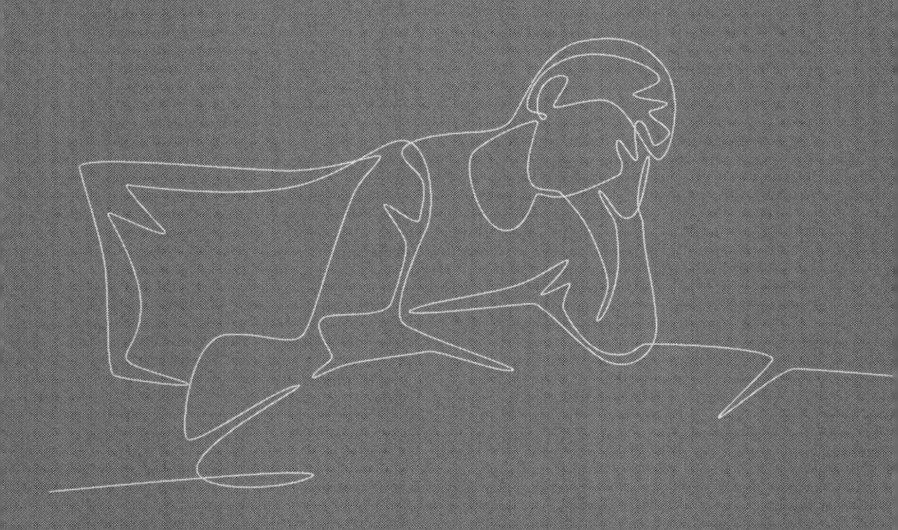

Stress and anxiety have become all too familiar companions in our modern world, often wreaking havoc on our mental and physical health. Left unchecked, these conditions can disrupt our sleep, affect our productivity, and reduce our quality of life. Fortunately, nature provides a wealth of calming herbs that can help us face life's challenges more gracefully. This chapter explores calming herbs for anxiety, natural sleep aids, and herbs that promote mental clarity and focus.

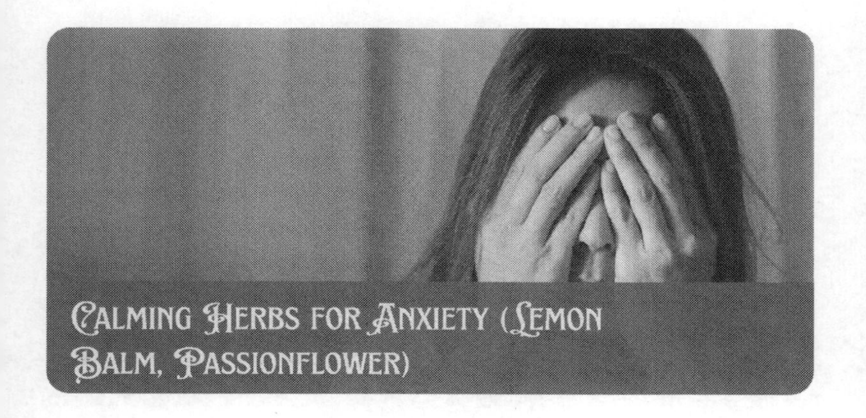

Calming Herbs for Anxiety (Lemon Balm, Passionflower)

Anxiety can feel overwhelming, but herbal medicine offers a gentle and effective way to restore balance to the nervous system. Using calming herbs is a holistic approach that not only relieves symptoms, but also nurtures the mind and body. Let's explore some of the most effective herbs for calming anxiety and promoting relaxation.

Lemon Balm (*Melissa officinalis*)

Lemon balm, a fragrant member of the mint family, has been valued for centuries for its calming and uplifting properties. Known for its gentle yet effective ability to reduce anxiety and improve mood, lemon balm works by increasing levels of gamma-aminobutyric acid (GABA) in the brain.

GABA is a neurotransmitter that inhibits nerve transmission and has a calming effect on the nervous system. Scientific studies have shown that lemon balm can help reduce symptoms of anxiety, promote a sense of well-being, and even improve cognitive function when stress levels are high.

How to use: Lemon balm can be enjoyed as a tea, tincture, or supplement. To make a soothing tea, steep 1-2 teaspoons of dried lemon balm leaves in a cup of hot water for 10-15 minutes. Drink this tea up to three times a day to experience its calming effects. Lemon balm tincture can also be taken in doses of 30-40 drops, up to three times a day, but consult a healthcare provider for personalized guidance.

Passionflower (*Passiflora incarnata*)

Passionflower is another remarkable herb that has been traditionally used to treat anxiety and insomnia. It is believed to increase the activity of GABA in the brain, which helps to calm the mind and relax the body. Passionflower has been studied for its effectiveness in reducing anxiety, and research suggests that it may be as effective as some prescription anti-anxiety medications, with fewer side effects. It is particularly helpful for those who experience anxiety-related sleep disturbances.

How to use: Passion flower can be consumed as a tea, tincture, or capsule. To make passion flower tea, steep 1-2 teaspoons of dried passion flower in a cup of hot water for 10 minutes. Drink this tea in the evening to relax and prepare for a restful sleep. A tincture of passion flower may be taken in doses of 20-40 drops, up to three times a day, depending on the severity of the anxiety. Always follow recommended guidelines and consult a healthcare professional as passion flower may interact with certain medications.

Chamomile (*Matricaria chamomilla*)

Chamomile is one of the best known and most widely used herbs for calming anxiety and promoting relaxation. It contains the flavonoid apigenin, which binds to benzodiazepine receptors in the brain, producing a mild sedative effect. Chamomile is effective in reducing symptoms of anxiety, calming the nervous system, and improving sleep quality. It is a gentle herb, making it suitable for both adults and children.

How to use: Chamomile is most commonly consumed as tea. To make chamomile tea, steep 1-2 tablespoons of dried chamomile flowers in a cup of boiling water for 5-10 minutes. Drink this tea before bed to relax and help you fall asleep, or during the day to calm your nerves. Chamomile can also be used in tincture form, with a typical dose of 20-30 drops taken up to three times a day. For skin conditions such as tension rashes or eczema, chamomile can be used topically as a soothing compress.

Lavender (*Lavandula angustifolia*)

Lavender is prized for its calming aroma and ability to reduce anxiety. It is often used in aromatherapy to promote relaxation and reduce stress. Lavender's calming effects are supported by research showing that inhaling lavender essential oil can lower heart rate and blood pressure, both of which are elevated during times of anxiety. The herb also has mild sedative effects, making it beneficial for people who struggle with sleep disturbances related to anxiety.

How to use: Lavender can be used in several forms, including tea, essential oil, or capsules. To make lavender tea, steep 1 teaspoon of dried lavender buds in hot water for 5-10 minutes. Drinking this tea can help reduce anxiety and promote relaxation. Lavender essential oil can be diffused in the air, added to a warm bath, or applied to pulse points (diluted with a carrier oil) for an immediate calming effect. Lavender capsules are available for those who prefer a more concentrated form, but always follow dosage instructions and seek professional advice if necessary.

Valerian Root (*Valeriana officinalis*)

Valerian root is a powerful herb often used to treat anxiety and promote restful sleep. It works by increasing GABA levels in the brain, similar to lemon balm and passion flower, but has a stronger sedative effect. Valerian is particularly useful for people who experience anxiety that interferes with their sleep. Studies have shown that valerian root can improve sleep quality and reduce the time it takes to fall asleep, making it a popular natural remedy for insomnia.

How to use: Valerian root can be taken as a tea, tincture, or capsule. To make valerian tea, steep 1 teaspoon of dried valerian root in a cup of hot water for 10-15 minutes. The tea has a strong and somewhat earthy flavor, so it may be mixed with other herbs, such as chamomile or lemon balm, to improve the taste. Valerian capsules or tinctures are also available, with dosages typically ranging from 300-600 mg before bed. Note that valerian should not be used long-term without professional guidance, and some people may experience drowsiness or vivid dreams as side effects.

These calming herbs offer a natural and holistic way to manage anxiety, reduce stress, and promote relaxation. By incorporating them into daily routines, individuals can experience a greater sense of well-being and balance.

However, it's important to consult with a healthcare professional to ensure that these herbs are safe and appropriate for your specific needs, especially if you are pregnant, nursing, or taking other medications.

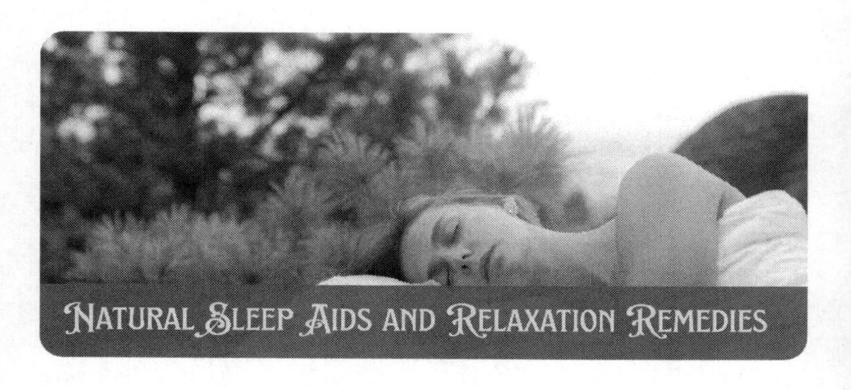

Natural Sleep Aids and Relaxation Remedies

Getting a good night's sleep is essential for both physical and emotional health. Unfortunately, stress, anxiety, and a fast-paced lifestyle often make it difficult to relax and get a good night's sleep. Fortunately, several herbs have been traditionally used to treat sleep disorders and promote relaxation. Let's explore some of the most effective natural sleep aids.

Ashwagandha (*Withania somnifera*)

Ashwagandha is a powerful adaptogenic herb known for its ability to help the body cope with stress. It works by lowering levels of cortisol, the hormone responsible for stress, and promoting a state of calm. Ashwagandha is particularly beneficial for improving sleep quality. Research has shown that it can help people fall asleep faster and experience deeper, more restorative sleep.

By regulating the hypothalamic-pituitary-adrenal (HPA) axis, ashwagandha reduces the stress response, allowing the body to relax and prepare for rest.

How to use: Ashwagandha is commonly available in powder, capsule, or tincture form. To make an ashwagandha sleep tonic, mix 1/2 to 1 teaspoon of ashwagandha powder into a glass of warm milk or a non-dairy alternative, adding a touch of honey for sweetness. Drink this an hour before bedtime to promote relaxation. For those who prefer capsules, a dose of 300-600 mg taken daily has been found to be effective. Always consult a health care professional before use, especially if you are pregnant, nursing, or have underlying health conditions.

Magnolia Bark (*Magnolia officinalis*)

Magnolia bark has been used in traditional Chinese medicine for thousands of years to treat anxiety and improve sleep. It contains bioactive compounds such as honokiol and magnolol, which have sedative properties. These compounds work by binding to GABA receptors in the brain, promoting relaxation and reducing the time it takes to fall asleep. Magnolia bark is especially helpful for people who experience sleep disturbances due to anxiety.

How to use: Magnolia bark can be taken as a tea, tincture, or supplement. To make a calming tea, steep 1 teaspoon of dried magnolia bark in hot water for 10-15 minutes. Drink this tea 30 minutes before bedtime to help you fall asleep. Magnolia bark supplements are also available in capsule form, but be sure to follow the recommended dosage on the product label.

Hops (*Humulus lupulus*)

Most people know hops as a key ingredient in beer, but they also have powerful sedative effects that can promote better sleep. Hops are often used in herbal medicine to treat insomnia and restlessness. They contain compounds that act on the central nervous system to reduce anxiety and promote a state of calm. Research has shown that hops can improve sleep quality, especially when combined with other sedative herbs such as valerian root.

How to use: Hops can be used in several forms, including tea, tinctures, and herbal pillows.

To make hop tea, steep 1-2 teaspoons of dried hop flowers in hot water for 10 minutes. Drink this tea in the evening to relax your body and prepare for a restful night's sleep. Herbal sleep pillows filled with hops and other calming herbs such as lavender and chamomile can also be placed near your pillow to create a soothing environment.

California Poppy (*Eschscholzia californica*)

California poppy is a mild, non-addictive sedative herb that can be used to treat mild anxiety and insomnia. It has a calming effect on the nervous system and can help you fall asleep without causing grogginess the next day. California poppy is especially beneficial for people who have trouble falling asleep due to racing thoughts or anxiety.

How to use: California poppy can be consumed as a tea, tincture, or capsule. To make a relaxing tea, steep 1-2 teaspoons of dried California poppy in a cup of hot water for 10 minutes. Drink this tea one hour before bedtime. Tinctures can be taken in doses of 20-30 drops before bedtime, but it is important to consult a healthcare professional for the appropriate dosage.

Skullcap (*Scutellaria lateriflora*)

Skullcap is a nervine herb known for its ability to calm an overactive mind and promote relaxation. It is especially helpful for people who have trouble sleeping due to stress or worry. Skullcap works by nourishing the nervous system and relieving tension, making it easier to drift off to sleep.

How to use: Skullcap can be made into a tea or taken as a tincture. To make skullcap tea, steep 1 teaspoon of dried skullcap in a cup of boiling water for 10 minutes. Drink this tea in the evening to relax and unwind. Skullcap tincture can also be taken in doses of 20-30 drops, up to three times a day, to reduce anxiety and promote restful sleep.

Incorporating these herbs into your bedtime routine can create a peaceful and relaxing environment conducive to sleep. Whether you choose to drink a warm herbal tea, use tinctures, or incorporate aromatherapy, these natural remedies can help improve your sleep quality and overall well-being.

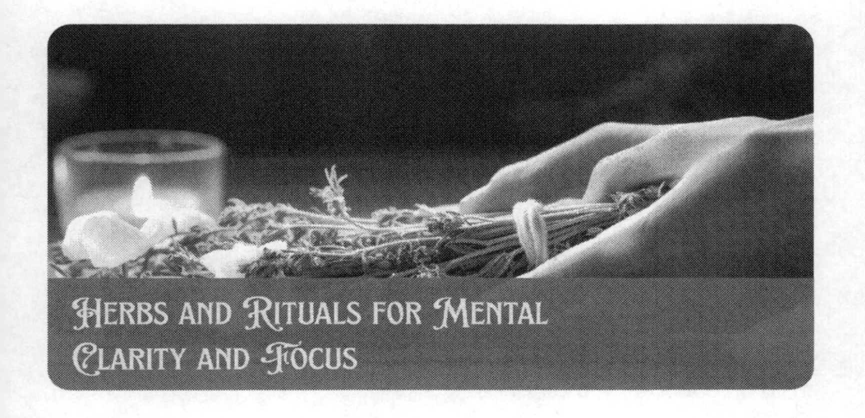

Herbs and Rituals for Mental Clarity and Focus

In a world full of distractions, maintaining mental clarity and focus can be a challenge. Cognitive health is affected by many factors, including stress, diet, and sleep quality. Fortunately, certain herbs can support brain function, improve concentration, and boost memory. Let's explore the best herbs for mental clarity and the rituals that can keep your mind sharp.

Ginkgo Biloba

Ginkgo biloba is one of the oldest living tree species and has been used in traditional medicine to improve cognitive function and memory. It works by increasing blood flow to the brain, which improves oxygen and nutrient delivery. Ginkgo biloba is also a powerful antioxidant that protects brain cells from damage caused by free radicals. Studies have shown that Ginkgo can improve mental performance and may even help prevent cognitive decline in older adults.

How to use: Ginkgo biloba is available in several forms, including capsules, tablets, and liquid extracts. The recommended dosage for cognitive support is typically 120-240 mg per day, divided into two or three doses. Be sure to consult with a healthcare provider before using ginkgo as it may interact with certain medications, especially blood thinners.

Rhodiola Rosea

Rhodiola rosea is an adaptogen that has been used for centuries to increase mental stamina and combat fatigue. It helps the body adapt to stress and can improve concentration and memory. Rhodiola is especially useful for people experiencing mental fog or burnout. By balancing stress hormones and supporting neurotransmitter function, Rhodiola improves cognitive performance and promotes mental clarity.

How to use: Rhodiola may be taken in capsule or tincture form. The typical dosage is 200-600 mg per day, taken in the morning or early afternoon. It is best to start with a lower dose and gradually increase it as needed. Rhodiola should not be taken late in the day as it may be stimulating and interfere with sleep.

Gotu Kola (*Centella asiatica*)

Gotu kola is often referred to as the "herb of longevity" in traditional medicine. It is known for its ability to improve cognitive function, enhance memory, and promote mental clarity. Gotu kola works by increasing blood flow and supporting the health of brain cells. It also has adaptogenic properties, making it useful for reducing stress and improving focus.

How to use: Gotu kola can be consumed as a tea, tincture, or capsule. To make gotu kola tea, steep 1 teaspoon of dried leaves in a cup of hot water for 10 minutes. Drinking this tea daily can support cognitive health. Gotu kola tincture can be taken in doses of 30-40 drops, up to three times a day, for improved focus and mental clarity.

Lion's Mane Mushroom (*Hericium erinaceus*)

Lion's mane is a unique medicinal mushroom that has been shown to support brain health and cognitive function. It contains compounds called hericenones and erinacines that stimulate the production of nerve growth factor (NGF). NGF is essential for the growth and maintenance of neurons, the cells responsible for transmitting information in the brain. Lion's Mane is known for its ability to improve memory, concentration, and overall mental clarity.

How to use: Lion's mane can be taken as a supplement, added to food, or consumed as a tea. The recommended dosage for cognitive support is 500-1,000 mg per day. Lion's mane powder can be added to smoothies, soups, or coffee for a brain-boosting effect. Be sure to choose high-quality lion's mane supplements from reputable sources.

Tulsi (*Ocimum sanctum*)

Tulsi, also known as holy basil, is an adaptogenic herb that can help clear mental fog and improve focus. It reduces stress hormones, increases cerebral blood flow, and supports overall brain function. Tulsi tea is commonly used in Ayurvedic medicine to promote mental clarity and emotional balance.

How to use: Tulsi can be consumed as tea or taken in capsule form. To make tulsi tea, steep 1-2 teaspoons of dried tulsi leaves in a cup of boiling water for 10 minutes. Drinking tulsi tea in the morning can help you feel alert and focused throughout the day. Tulsi capsules can be taken as directed, but consult a healthcare provider to determine the best dosage for your needs.

Rituals for Mental Clarity

In addition to herbal remedies, incorporating daily rituals can help maintain mental sharpness and focus. These rituals include

Mindfulness meditation: Practicing mindfulness meditation for 10-20 minutes a day can improve focus and reduce mental clutter. It trains the mind to stay present, which improves cognitive performance.

Regular physical activity: Exercise increases blood flow to the brain and releases endorphins, which boost mood and improve cognitive function. Aim for at least 30 minutes of moderate activity most days of the week.

Get enough sleep: Prioritizing sleep is critical for mental clarity. Establish a consistent sleep schedule and bedtime routine to ensure you get 7-9 hours of quality sleep each night.

Eat a brain-boosting diet: A diet rich in antioxidants, healthy fats, and vitamins can support brain health. Foods such as leafy greens, nuts, seeds, and fatty fish are especially beneficial.

By incorporating these herbs and rituals into your daily routine, you can naturally support mental clarity and focus, increase productivity, and improve your overall well-being. Always consult a health care professional before starting any new herbal regimen to ensure it is appropriate for your health needs.

BOOK 02

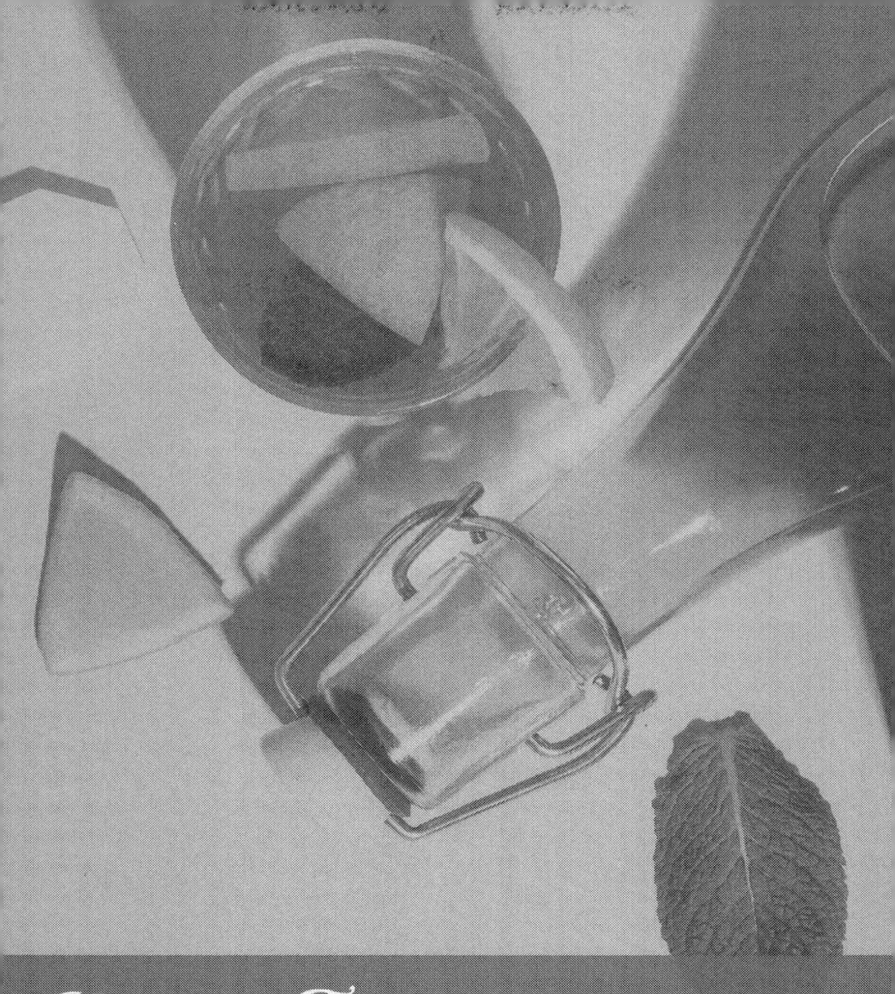

Herbal Teas and Glycerin or Vinegar-Based Tinctures for Vitality and Wellness

CHAPTER 1

Introduction to Medicinal Teas and Their Benefits

Herbal teas have been treasured for centuries as a natural way to promote wellness, offering a range of health benefits through the careful infusion of herbs. Unlike traditional tea made from the *Camellia sinensis* plant, herbal teas, also known as tisanes, are made by steeping various parts of the plant, such as leaves, flowers, roots, seeds, or bark. The simple act of brewing herbal tea not only releases the therapeutic properties of the herbs, but also provides a soothing ritual that can be incorporated into daily life. In this chapter, we will explore the art and science of blending herbs for tea, the best times to consume different herbal teas, and how to select herbs based on their energetic properties to create truly personalized and effective infusions.

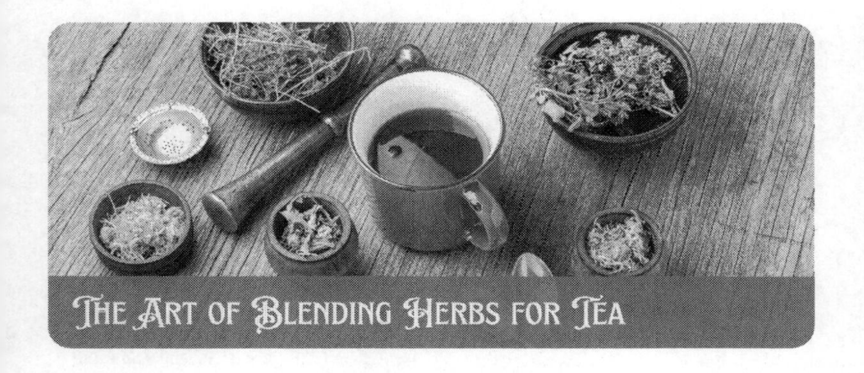

The Art of Blending Herbs for Tea

Blending herbs for tea is both an art and a science. The goal is to create a balanced infusion that is not only medically beneficial, but also pleasing to the senses. A well-crafted herbal blend takes into account the flavor, aroma, color, and therapeutic properties of each ingredient. Mastering the art of herbal blending can transform a simple cup of tea into a powerful healing experience.

Understanding the Basics of Herbal Blending

When creating an herbal tea blend, it is important to think about the role each herb will play in the blend. In general, the herbs in a blend fall into three main categories:

Base herbs (main ingredient): These are the primary herbs that make up the bulk of the blend, typically making up about 50-70% of the mixture. Base herbs tend to be mild in flavor and have broad-spectrum benefits. Examples include *Rooibos* for a caffeine-free antioxidant boost or *Nettle* for its nourishing and mineral-rich properties.

Supporting Herbs (Secondary Ingredients): These herbs complement the base herbs and enhance the therapeutic effects of the tea. They typically make up 20-30% of the blend. Supporting herbs often target specific body systems. For example, *Peppermint* may be added to support digestion, while *Elderflower* may be used to strengthen the immune system.

Accent Herbs (Flavor and Aroma Enhancers): These herbs add flavor, aroma and sometimes a pop of color to the tea. They make up about 10-20% of the blend and ensure that the tea is pleasant to drink. Common accent herbs include *Lavender*, *Hibiscus*, *Rose Petals*, and *Cinnamon*.

Choosing the Right Ingredients

Creating an effective herbal tea blend begins with selecting high-quality, organic herbs. Freshly dried herbs retain more of their medicinal properties than herbs that have been stored for a long time. The potency of herbs should be judged by their vibrant color and strong aroma. Whenever possible, use locally grown herbs to ensure freshness.

Flavor Balance: Achieving the right balance of flavors is critical. Herbs can be categorized as sweet (e.g., *Licorice Root*), bitter (e.g., *Dandelion Root*), spicy (e.g., *Ginger*), sour (e.g., *Hibiscus*), or earthy (e.g., *Burdock Root*). Combining different flavor profiles can make the tea more enjoyable. For example, a digestive blend might include bitter dandelion root to stimulate digestion, sweet licorice root to balance the bitterness, and spicy ginger to add warmth.

Therapeutic Intent: Consider the desired therapeutic outcome of the blend. Is the goal to calm the mind, support the immune system, or increase energy levels? Tailor the blend to address specific health concerns while keeping in mind the overall harmony of the herbs. For example, a calming tea for stress relief might include *Lemon Balm*, *Chamomile*, and a touch of *Rose Petals* for a soothing experience.

Blending Techniques

There are two primary methods for blending herbs:

Dry Blending: This method involves measuring and mixing dried herbs in a large bowl. Once mixed, the mixture should be stored in an airtight container away from light and heat. Label the container with the name of the blend and the date it was made to keep track of freshness. Dry blending is ideal for making larger batches that can be enjoyed over time.

Infusion Blending: This method involves steeping individual herbs separately and then combining the liquid extracts. Infusion blending allows for greater control over the strength and flavor of each herb in the tea. It is especially useful when working with herbs that have a strong or bitter taste.

Experimenting and Adjusting

Blending herbal teas is a creative process that often requires experimentation. Start with small batches to test your blend and make adjustments as needed. Keep a journal to record the proportions and effects of different herbs, as this will help you refine your technique over time. Be open to experimenting with new combinations, but always make sure that the herbs you use are safe and appropriate for their intended use.

Sample Herbal Tea Blends

To get you started, here are a few sample blends:

1. **Calm and relax tea:** *Lemon Balm* (base), *Oatstraw* (support), *Lavender* (accent)
2. **Immune-boosting blend:** *Echinacea* (base), *Elderflower* (support), *Orange Peel* (accent)
3. **Digestive Comfort Tea:** *Peppermint* (base), *Fennel* (support), *Calendula* (accent).

These blends can be enjoyed daily or used as needed to support specific health goals. Remember, the best herbal tea blend is one that meets your individual needs and tastes great.

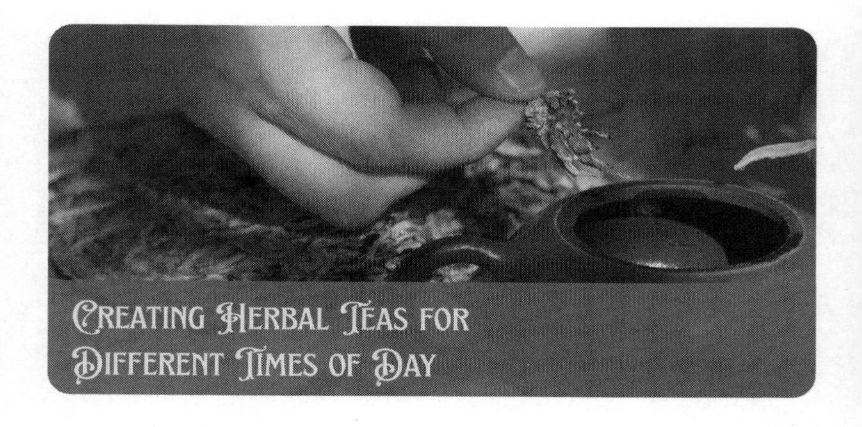

Creating Herbal Teas for Different Times of Day

Herbal teas can be tailored to different times of the day to maximize their benefits and fit seamlessly into your daily routine. By choosing specific herbs that align with your body's natural rhythms, you can create a series of teas that energize you in the morning, sustain you through the afternoon, and soothe you into a restful evening. Understanding the properties of different herbs and how they affect your energy and focus can transform the way you experience your day.

Morning Teas: Energizing and Uplifting

Morning is a time for energizing herbs that wake up the body and mind without the jitters of caffeine. The goal is to use herbs that gently increase energy levels, improve mental clarity, and prepare the body for the day ahead.

Peppermint *(Mentha piperita)*: A refreshing and invigorating herb, peppermint is known to stimulate the senses and promote mental alertness. The menthol in peppermint provides a natural energy boost and helps clear brain fog. It is an excellent choice for starting the day with a clear mind.

Holy Basil *(Tulsi) (Ocimum sanctum):* Holy basil is revered in Ayurvedic medicine for its adaptogenic properties, which help the body adapt to stress while providing a gentle energy boost. Drinking tulsi tea in the morning can set a positive tone for the day and support overall well-being.

Ginseng ***(Panax ginseng or Eleutherococcus senticosus)*****:** Both types of ginseng are known for their ability to increase stamina and reduce fatigue. Siberian ginseng (Eleuthero) is particularly good for improving physical endurance and mental performance.

Lemongrass ***(Cymbopogon citratus)*****:** With its bright, citrusy flavor, lemongrass tea is uplifting and helps awaken the senses. It also has digestive benefits, making it an excellent morning tea to enjoy with breakfast.

Morning Tea Recipe:

- 1 teaspoon peppermint leaves
- 1 teaspoon holy basil leaves
- 1/2 teaspoon lemongrass
- Steep in hot water for 5–7 minutes, strain, and enjoy to kickstart your day.

Afternoon Teas: Rejuvenating and Balancing

The afternoon is often when energy levels begin to wane, making it the perfect time to turn to herbs that offer gentle rejuvenation. Afternoon teas should provide sustained energy and focus without interfering with the natural winding down process that occurs in the evening.

Rooibos ***(Aspalathus linearis)*****:** Rooibos is a naturally caffeine-free tea that is rich in antioxidants. It provides a mild energy boost without overstimulating the nervous system and is known for its earthy, slightly sweet flavor.

Ginger ***(Zingiber officinale)*****:** Ginger is warming and invigorating, making it ideal for digestion and boosting energy in the afternoon. It also helps improve circulation, which can be beneficial if you've been sitting for a long time.

Spearmint ***(Mentha spicata)*****:** Similar to peppermint but milder, spearmint provides a refreshing pick-me-up while aiding digestion. It's a great herb to combine with rooibos for a flavorful afternoon tea.

Ashwagandha ***(Withania somnifera)*****:** An adaptogenic herb that helps the body manage stress and maintain energy, ashwagandha can provide a sense of calm focus, making it ideal for afternoon tea.

Afternoon Tea Recipe:

- 1 tablespoon rooibos
- 1/2 teaspoon ginger root
- 1 teaspoon spearmint
- 1/2 teaspoon ashwagandha powder
- Steep in hot water for 7–10 minutes, strain, and enjoy to rejuvenate your afternoon.

Evening Teas: Calming and Relaxing

Evening teas should be designed to calm the mind, relax the body, and prepare you for a restful night's sleep. These teas focus on using herbs with mild sedative effects that promote relaxation and support the natural sleep cycle.

Chamomile *(Matricaria chamomilla)*: Chamomile is one of the most well-known herbs for relaxation. It calms the nervous system and helps reduce anxiety, making it perfect for unwinding in the evening.

Skullcap *(Scutellaria lateriflora)*: This nervine herb is excellent for calming an overactive mind. It is especially useful for people who have difficulty letting go of stress and worry before bedtime.

Hops *(Humulus lupulus)*: Hops are often used to promote sleep and relaxation. The sedative compounds in hops work well in combination with other calming herbs to enhance their effects.

Pau d'Arco *(Tabebuia impetiginosa)*: Lemon verbena is calming and has a delightful citrus flavor that blends well with other calming herbs. It helps relax the body and mind, preparing you for a restful night's sleep.

Evening Tea Recipe:

- 1 teaspoon chamomile flowers
- 1/2 teaspoon skullcap
- 1/2 teaspoon hops
- 1/2 teaspoon lemon verbena
- Steep in hot water for 5–7 minutes, strain, and sip slowly to unwind.

These herbal tea recipes are designed to fit into different parts of your day, supporting your body's natural rhythms and enhancing your overall sense of well-being.

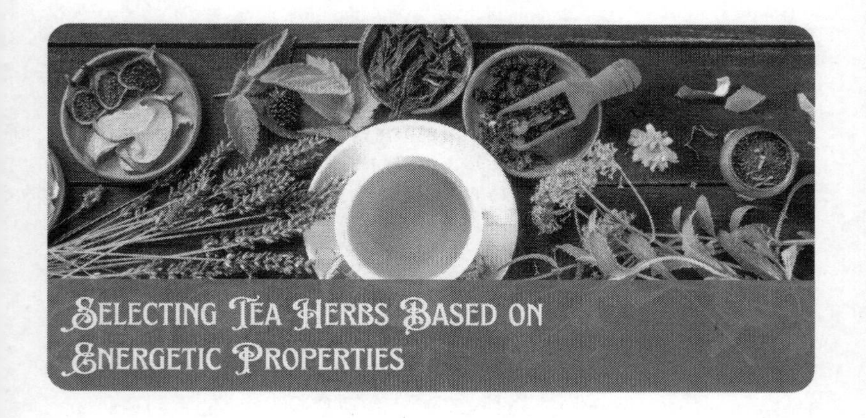

Selecting Tea Herbs Based on Energetic Properties

Herbs have unique energetic properties that can influence how they affect the body. In traditional healing systems such as Ayurveda and Traditional Chinese Medicine (TCM), the energetics of an herb are considered as important as its chemical constituents. Understanding the warming, cooling, moisturizing, or drying properties of herbs can help you choose the right ones to support balance in your body.

Understanding Herb Energetics

The energetic properties of herbs are often described in terms of temperature (warming or cooling), moisture (moisturizing or drying), and action (stimulating or calming). By considering these qualities, you can create tea blends that address specific imbalances or support your body's natural constitution.

Warming herbs: These herbs increase circulation, raise body temperature, and are often used to combat cold conditions. Examples include *Ginger*, *Cinnamon*, and *Clove*. Warming herbs are especially helpful during the colder months or for people who naturally feel cold or sluggish.

Cooling herbs: These herbs reduce inflammation, calm the nervous system, and lower body temperature. Examples include *Peppermint*, *Spearmint*, and *Hibiscus*. Cooling herbs are ideal for hot climates, fevers, or people who tend to run hot.

Moisturizing herbs: These herbs help hydrate tissues and are used for conditions associated with dryness, such as dry skin or a dry throat. Examples include *Marshmallow Root*, *Licorice Root*, and *Oatstraw*. Moisturizing herbs are especially useful during dry seasons or for people who are prone to dehydration.

Dehydrating herbs: These herbs help remove excess moisture from the body and are useful for conditions such as congestion or edema. Examples include *Sage*, *Thyme*, and *Nettle*. Drying herbs are beneficial for people who are prone to moisture or mucus buildup.

Matching Herbs to Your Constitution

In traditional medicine, understanding your constitution-whether you are naturally hot, cold, dry, or humid-can guide your choice of herbs. Here's how to approach herbal selection based on your body's energetic needs:

For Cold Constitutions (Tend to Feel Cold and Lethargic)

- Opt for warming herbs like *Ginger*, *Cinnamon*, and *Black Pepper*.
- These herbs can help boost circulation and energy levels, making you feel warmer and more invigorated.

For Hot Constitutions (Tend to Feel Overheated and Irritable)

- Choose cooling herbs such as *Peppermint*, *Hibiscus*, and *Chamomile*.
- These herbs help reduce inflammation, calm the mind, and cool down the body.

For Dry Constitutions (Prone to Dry Skin, Throat, or Lungs)

- Use moistening herbs like *Marshmallow Root*, *Slippery Elm*, and *Oatstraw*.
- These herbs provide hydration and soothe irritated tissues, making them ideal for dry conditions.

For Moist Constitutions (Experience Excess Mucus or Fluid Retention)

- Go for drying herbs like *Sage*, *Thyme*, and *Nettle*.
- These herbs help remove excess moisture and reduce congestion, promoting balance.

Creating Energetic Tea Blends

When creating energetic tea blends, consider the season, your current health, and your body's natural tendencies. For example, in the winter, a warming blend with *Cinnamon* and *Ginger* may help increase circulation, while in the summer, a cooling blend with *Peppermint* and *Hibiscus* may be more appropriate.

Sample Energetic Tea Blends:

- **Winter Warming Blend:** *Cinnamon*, *Ginger*, *Cardamom*
- **Summer Cooling Blend:** *Hibiscus*, *Peppermint*, *Lemon Balm*
- **Dry Skin Soother:** *Marshmallow Root*, *Oatstraw*, *Calendula*
- **Congestion Relief Tea:** *Sage*, *Thyme*, *Elderflower*

By understanding the energetic properties of herbs and how they interact with your body, you can create personalized

CHAPTER 2

Non-Alcohol Tinctures for Targeted Health Support

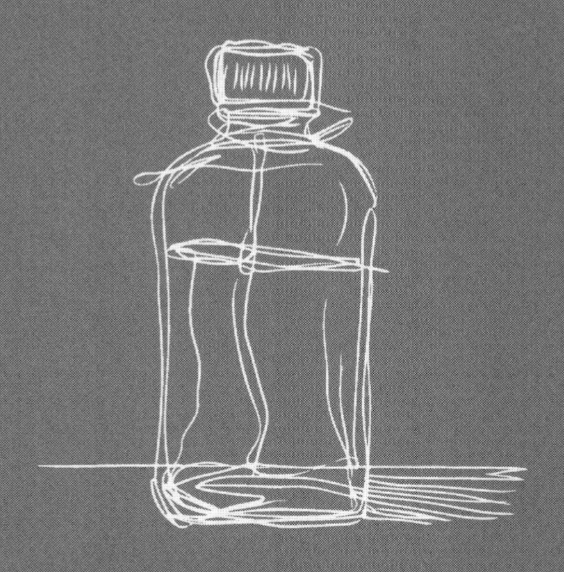

In herbal medicine, tinctures are concentrated extracts that capture the therapeutic properties of herbs. Traditionally, alcohol has been used as a solvent in tincture preparation due to its effectiveness in extracting a wide range of plant constituents. However, for individuals seeking alcohol-free alternatives-whether for health, personal, or religious reasons-glycerin and vinegar offer viable substitutes. These non-alcoholic tinctures, known as glycerin and vinegar-based tinctures, provide a gentle yet effective means of harnessing the benefits of herbs.

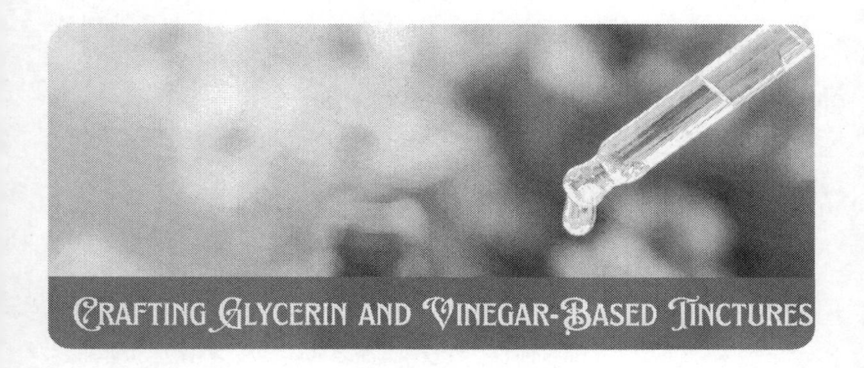

Crafting Glycerin and Vinegar-Based Tinctures

Creating glycerin and vinegar-based tinctures requires selecting appropriate herbs, understanding the properties of each solvent, and following meticulous preparation methods to ensure potency and safety.

Glycerin-Based Tinctures (Glycerites):

Vegetable glycerin, a sweet tasting syrupy liquid derived from plant oils, is an excellent solvent for extracting certain herbal constituents. Glycerin is preferred for its palatability, making it suitable for children and those sensitive to alcohol.

Preparation Steps:

Selecting Herbs: Choose dried herbs, as fresh herbs contain water that can dilute the glycerin and potentially cause spoilage.

Diluting Glycerin: For optimal extraction, dilute glycerin with distilled water at a ratio of 3:1 (three parts glycerin to one part water).

Combining Ingredients: Place the dried herbs in a sterilized glass jar, filling it about halfway. Pour the diluted glycerin over the herbs, making sure they are completely submerged.

Maceration process: Seal jar tightly and store in a cool, dark place. Shake the jar daily to facilitate extraction. Allow the mixture to macerate for 4 to 6 weeks.

Straining and Storage: After the maceration period, strain the liquid through a fine mesh strainer or cheesecloth into a clean jar. Store the glycerol in a dark glass bottle away from direct sunlight.

Vinegar-Based Tinctures:

Apple cider vinegar (ACV) is a popular solvent for making non-alcoholic tinctures. Its acidic nature effectively extracts minerals and alkaloids from herbs, and it offers additional health benefits such as aiding digestion and supporting the immune system.

Preparation Steps:

Select herbs: Both fresh and dried herbs can be used. If using fresh herbs, make sure they are clean and free of moisture to prevent mold growth.

Combine ingredients: Fill a sterilized glass jar two-thirds full with fresh herbs or one-third full with dried herbs. Pour raw, unfiltered apple cider vinegar over the herbs, leaving about an inch of space at the top.

Macerate: Cover the jar with a plastic lid or place a piece of wax paper between the metal lid and the jar to prevent corrosion. Store the jar in a cool, dark place and shake daily. Allow to macerate for 4 to 6 weeks.

Straining and storage: After the maceration period, strain the liquid through cheesecloth into a clean jar. Store the vinegar-based tincture in a dark glass bottle away from direct sunlight.

Considerations:

Shelf Life: Glycerites typically have a shelf life of 1 to 2 years when properly stored, while vinegar-based tinctures can last up to a year.

Dosage: Non-alcoholic tinctures are generally taken in slightly larger doses than alcohol-based tinctures. A common dosage is 1 to 2 teaspoons up to three times daily, but it's important to consult with a healthcare professional for personalized guidance.

Storage: Always store tinctures in dark glass bottles to protect them from light, which can reduce their potency. Store them in a cool, dark place and make sure the bottles are tightly sealed to prevent oxidation.

By using glycerin and vinegar as solvents, individuals can create effective, alcohol-free tinctures tailored to their health needs, ensuring accessibility and inclusivity in herbal medicine practices.

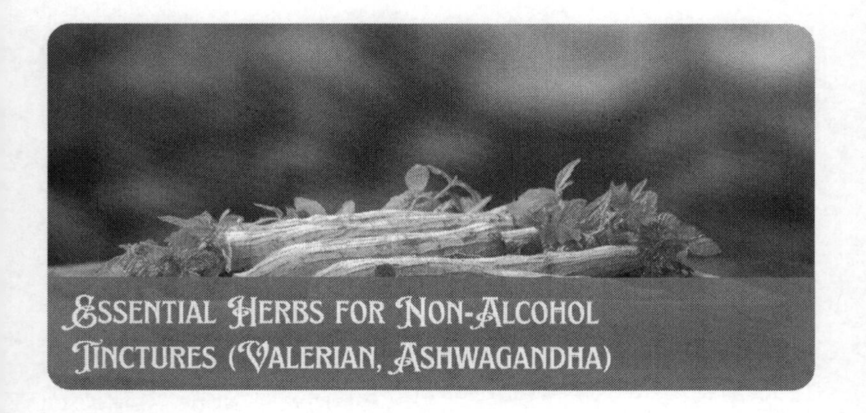

Essential Herbs for Non-Alcohol Tinctures (Valerian, Ashwagandha)

Creating effective non-alcoholic tinctures requires selecting herbs that are not only potent, but also well suited to the glycerin or vinegar extraction process. Valerian and ashwagandha are two herbs that are particularly well suited to this method, offering a range of therapeutic benefits without the use of alcohol.

Valerian (*Valeriana officinalis*)

Valerian root is known for its calming properties, making it a popular natural remedy for anxiety, insomnia, and muscle tension. The herb works by increasing the activity of gamma-aminobutyric acid (GABA) in the brain, which helps to calm the nervous system.

Primary Benefits:

- ***Sleep Support:*** Valerian is often used as a natural sleep aid to help those who have trouble falling asleep or staying asleep. It promotes deep, restful sleep without the grogginess often associated with pharmaceutical sedatives.
- ***Anxiety and Stress Relief:*** Valerian helps relieve anxiety and nervous tension, making it ideal for daytime use in small doses to calm an overactive mind.
- ***Muscle Relaxation:*** Valerian's antispasmodic properties make it useful for relieving muscle spasms, menstrual cramps, and tension headaches.

How to Use Valerian in a Glycerin-Based Tincture:

- ***Ingredients:*** Dried valerian root, vegetable glycerin, distilled water.
- ***Method:*** Chop the dried valerian root and fill a sterilized glass jar about one-third full. Mix three parts glycerin with one part distilled water and pour over the valerian until completely submerged. Seal the jar and store in a cool, dark place for 4 to 6 weeks, shaking gently each day. Strain the liquid and store in a dark glass bottle.

Ashwagandha (*Withania somnifera*)

Ashwagandha is a powerful adaptogen that has been used in Ayurvedic medicine for thousands of years. It helps the body manage stress, improve energy levels, and support overall well-being. The active ingredients, known as withanolides, have been shown to reduce cortisol levels, promote mental clarity, and support a balanced immune response.

Primary Benefits:

- ***Stress Reduction:*** Ashwagandha's adaptogenic properties help lower cortisol levels, reducing the effects of stress on the body and mind.
- ***Enhanced Mental Clarity:*** It supports brain function, improving focus, memory, and overall cognitive performance.
- ***Energy and vitality:*** Ashwagandha helps combat fatigue and supports sustained energy throughout the day without overstimulation.

How to Use Ashwagandha in a Vinegar-Based Tincture:

- ***Ingredients:*** Dried ashwagandha root, raw apple cider vinegar.
- ***Method:*** Place chopped ashwagandha root in a sterilized jar about one-third full. Cover with raw, unpasteurized apple cider vinegar, making sure the root is completely submerged. Place a piece of waxed paper under the lid to prevent corrosion and seal tightly. Let the mixture sit for 4 to 6 weeks, shaking the jar daily. Strain and store in a dark glass bottle.

Both of these herbs are versatile and effective when used in non-alcohol tinctures, offering a gentle way to support stress management, sleep, and overall vitality.

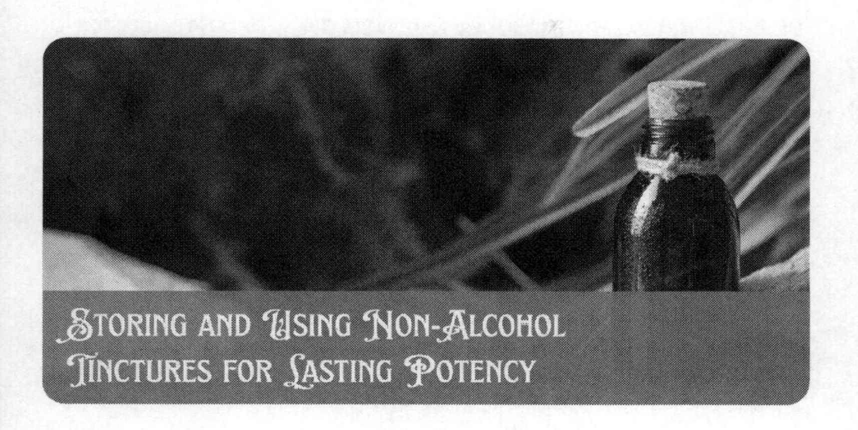

Storing and Using Non-Alcohol Tinctures for Lasting Potency

Proper storage and use of non-alcoholic tinctures is essential to maintain their potency and ensure their therapeutic efficacy. Glycerin and vinegar-based tinctures are more sensitive to environmental factors than their alcohol-based counterparts, so special care must be taken.

Storage Tips for Longevity

Use dark glass bottles: Store tinctures in amber or cobalt blue glass bottles to protect them from light, which can degrade the active compounds in the herbs. Exposure to light accelerates oxidation and shortens the shelf life of the tincture.

Cool, dark storage area: Store tinctures in a cool, dark place, such as a pantry or closet, away from direct sunlight and heat sources. Temperature fluctuations can affect the quality of the tincture.

Proper Sealing: Make sure bottles are tightly sealed to prevent air and moisture from entering. Exposure to air can cause oxidation and bacterial growth, especially in vinegar-based tinctures.

Labeling: Always label each tincture with the name of the herb(s), the solvent used, and the date it was made. This will help you keep track of the age of the tincture and ensure that you use it before it loses potency.

Shelf Life Considerations

Glycerin-based tinctures: These tinctures typically have a shelf life of 1 to 2 years when properly stored. The sweet taste of glycerin makes them appealing to children, but care should be taken to monitor for any changes in odor, color, or consistency that may indicate spoilage.

Vinegar-based tinctures: Vinegar-based tinctures generally last about 1 year. Vinegar acts as a preservative but is less effective than alcohol at preventing microbial growth. Check regularly for signs of spoilage, such as mold or a change in odor.

How to Use Non-Alcohol Tinctures

Dosage: The typical dosage for glycerin-based tinctures is 1 to 2 teaspoons, up to three times a day. Vinegar-based tinctures are usually taken in slightly smaller doses. Always consult a healthcare provider for personalized dosage recommendations, especially if you are pregnant, nursing, or taking medications.

Methods of administration: Non-alcoholic tinctures can be taken directly or diluted in a small amount of water, juice, or herbal tea. Their pleasant taste makes them easier to consume, especially for children and those who dislike the harshness of alcohol-based extracts.

Uses: Glycerin and vinegar tinctures can also be used topically for certain conditions. For example, a diluted vinegar tincture can be applied to the skin to soothe minor irritations or used as a compress for muscle aches.

By following these guidelines for storage and use, you can ensure that your alcohol-free tinctures remain effective and safe to use. These non-alcoholic options provide an accessible way to incorporate the healing power of herbs into daily wellness routines and cater to a wide range of preferences and needs.

CHAPTER 3

Herbal Teas and Tinctures for Energy and Vitality

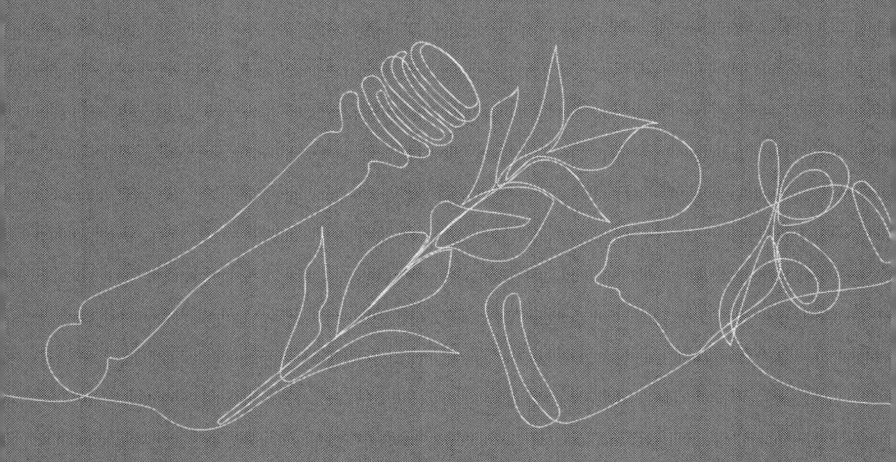

The fast pace of modern life often leaves us feeling drained and tired. Instead of relying on caffeine or artificial energy boosters that can cause a crash, herbal teas and tinctures offer a natural and sustainable way to boost energy and vitality. This chapter looks at specific herbs known for their revitalizing properties and how to use them in teas and tinctures for lasting, balanced energy.

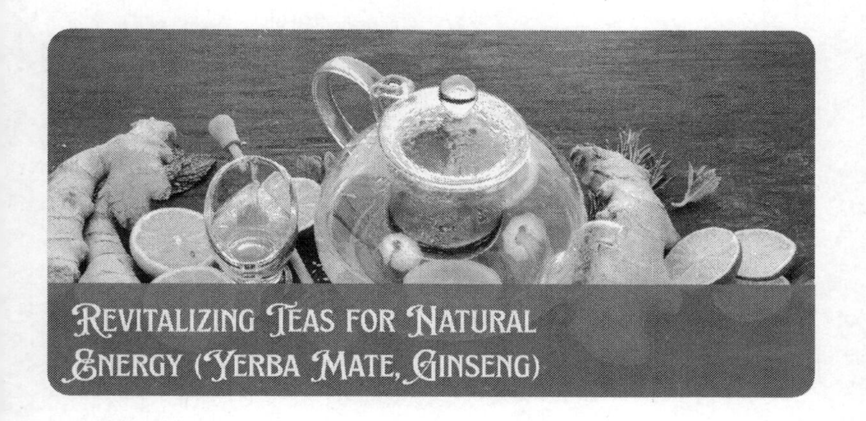

Revitalizing Teas for Natural Energy (Yerba Mate, Ginseng)

Herbal teas for energy are designed to provide a natural boost that improves mental clarity, physical stamina, and overall vitality without the side effects of stimulants like coffee. Yerba mate and ginseng stand out as two powerful herbs in this category, offering a variety of benefits for those looking to stay energized and focused throughout the day.

Yerba Mate (*Ilex paraguariensis*)

Yerba Mate, a traditional South American tea, has gained worldwide recognition for its energy-boosting properties. It contains a unique combination of caffeine, theobromine, and theophylline that work synergistically to provide a balanced, smooth energy boost. Unlike coffee, which often causes jitters and crashes, yerba mate provides sustained alertness and mental clarity.

Primary Benefits:

- ***Sustained Energy:*** The caffeine in Yerba Mate stimulates the central nervous system, enhancing focus and reducing fatigue without causing anxiety or restlessness.
- ***Rich in Antioxidants:*** Yerba Mate contains a high concentration of antioxidants, such as polyphenols and saponins, which support immune health and reduce inflammation.
- ***Digestive Aid:*** Yerba Mate can also aid digestion, making

it a well-rounded option for promoting overall wellness.

How to Prepare Yerba Mate Tea:

- ***Traditional Method:*** Yerba Mate is traditionally prepared in a gourd and sipped through a metal straw called a bombilla. The leaves are steeped in hot (not boiling) water to preserve the delicate compounds.
- ***Modern Brewing:*** For a simpler approach, use a tea infuser or French press. Steep 1 to 2 teaspoons of yerba mate leaves in hot (not boiling) water for 3 to 5 minutes. Sweeten with honey or add a squeeze of lemon juice if desired.

Ginseng (Panax ginseng and Eleutherococcus senticosus)

Ginseng is a well-known adaptogen that has been used in traditional medicine for centuries to increase energy, improve mental function, and strengthen the immune system. Both Panax ginseng (Asian ginseng) and Eleuthero (Siberian ginseng) have unique properties that make them powerful natural energizers.

Primary Benefits:

- ***Panax Ginseng (Asian Ginseng):*** Known for its powerful energy-boosting effects, Panax Ginseng improves physical performance, reduces fatigue, and supports cognitive function. It is particularly useful for those who experience mental fatigue or need to improve stamina.
- ***Eleuthero (Siberian Ginseng):*** Eleuthero is a mild adaptogen that helps the body adapt to stress and promotes overall vitality. It is ideal for long-term use to support sustained energy levels and improve the body's resilience to stress.

How to Prepare Ginseng Tea:

- ***Ingredients:*** Sliced ginseng root or powdered ginseng, hot water, and optional honey for sweetness.
- ***Method:*** Steep 1 to 2 slices of dried ginseng root or 1/2 teaspoon of powdered ginseng in hot water for 10 to 15 minutes. Strain and enjoy. For added flavor, consider blending with a mild herb such as peppermint or lemongrass.

Blending Yerba Mate and Ginseng for Maximum Impact

The combination of Yerba Mate and Ginseng creates a powerful tea blend that can provide both immediate and sustained energy. The stimulating effects of yerba mate complement the adaptogenic properties of ginseng, resulting in a balanced and effective energy boost.

Sample Recipe:

- 1 teaspoon Yerba Mate leaves
- 1 slice of dried Panax Ginseng or 1/2 teaspoon of Eleuthero root
- 1/2 teaspoon dried peppermint (optional for flavor)
- Steep in hot water for 5 to 7 minutes, strain, and enjoy.

This revitalizing blend can be enjoyed in the morning or early afternoon to support productivity and maintain energy levels throughout the day. In the next section, we will explore how to make anti-fatigue and endurance tinctures, providing additional tools for natural energy support.

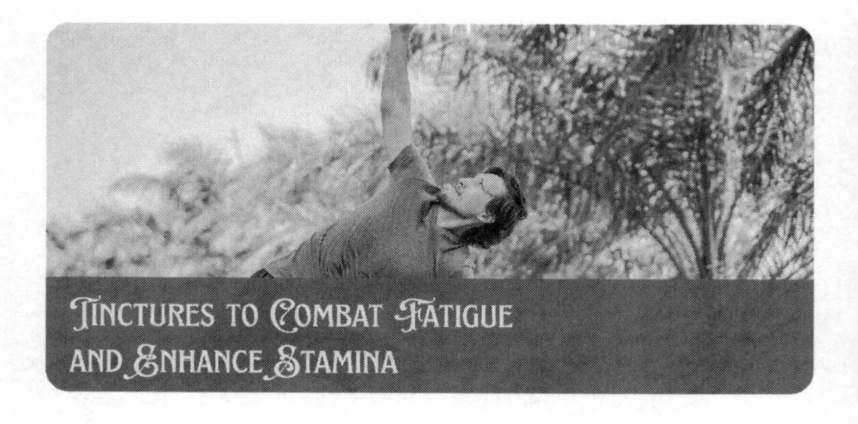

Tinctures to Combat Fatigue and Enhance Stamina

For those looking for a long-lasting, convenient way to enjoy the energizing effects of herbs, tinctures are an excellent option. Unlike teas, tinctures are concentrated extracts that are easy to carry and use throughout the day. This section focuses on creating tinctures using herbs known to combat fatigue and increase stamina, such as eleuthero, rhodiola, and maca.

Eleuthero *(Eleutherococcus senticosus)*

Eleuthero, also known as Siberian Ginseng, is an adaptogen that supports the body's ability to handle stress, increases energy levels, and improves physical performance. It is especially useful for athletes or those who need sustained energy throughout the day.

Primary Benefits:

- ***Stress Adaptation:*** Eleuthero helps balance cortisol levels, reducing the impact of stress on the body and promoting a steady flow of energy.
- ***Endurance and Stamina:*** It increases oxygen utilization and endurance, making it ideal for physical and mental exertion.
- ***Immune Support:*** Eleuthero also supports the immune system, making it a well-rounded herb for energy and vitality.

How to Make Eleuthero Tincture:

- ***Ingredients:*** Dried eleuthero root, vegetable glycerin, or apple cider vinegar.

- ***Method:*** Fill a sterilized jar one-third full with chopped dried eleuthero root. Cover with glycerin or vinegar, leaving an inch of space at the top. Seal tightly and store in a cool, dark place for 4 to 6 weeks, shaking daily. Strain and store in a dark glass bottle.
- *Take 1 to 2 teaspoons of eleuthero tincture up to twice daily. Always consult a healthcare provider for personalized advice, especially if pregnant or taking medications.*

Rhodiola (*Rhodiola rosea*)

Rhodiola is a powerful adaptogen known for its ability to reduce fatigue and increase physical and mental performance. It works by balancing neurotransmitters in the brain and supporting adrenal function.

Primary Benefits:

- ***Mental Clarity:*** Rhodiola helps improve concentration and reduce brain fog, making it ideal for students or professionals.
- ***Physical Stamina:*** It increases energy production at the cellular level, which increases stamina and reduces feelings of exhaustion.
- ***Mood Improvement:*** Rhodiola has mood-stabilizing effects, helping to alleviate mild depression and anxiety that are often associated with fatigue.

How to Make Rhodiola Tincture:

- ***Ingredients:***Dried Rhodiola root, vegetable glycerin, or apple cider vinegar.
- ***Method:*** Chop the dried Rhodiola root and place it in a sterilized jar, filling it one-third of the way. Pour the glycerin or vinegar over the root until completely submerged. Seal the jar and store in a cool, dark place, shaking daily, for 4 to 6 weeks. Strain and store in a dark glass bottle.
- ***Dosage:*** Take 1 to 2 teaspoons daily, preferably in the morning or early afternoon to avoid disturbing sleep.

Maca (*Lepidium meyenii*)

Maca root is a Peruvian superfood known for its ability to increase energy, stamina, and libido. It is rich in vitamins, minerals, and phytonutrients that nourish the body and support overall vitality.

Primary Benefits:

- ***Hormonal Balance:*** Maca is known to balance hormones, which can increase energy levels and improve mood.
- ***Physical Strength:*** It increases physical stamina and endurance, making it popular with athletes.
- ***Cognitive Function:*** Maca supports brain health and mental clarity, providing a well-rounded energy boost.

How to Make Maca Tincture:

- ***Ingredients:*** Dried Maca root powder, vegetable glycerin or apple cider vinegar.
- ***Directions:*** Mix 1 part Maca root powder with 3 parts glycerin or vinegar in a sterilized glass jar. Seal the jar and store in a cool, dark place, shaking daily for 4 weeks. Strain and store in a dark glass bottle.
- ***Dosage:*** Take 1 to 2 teaspoons daily. Maca tincture can be added to smoothies or taken directly.

These tinctures are a convenient way to combat fatigue and enhance stamina, providing a concentrated dose of herbal goodness whenever needed.

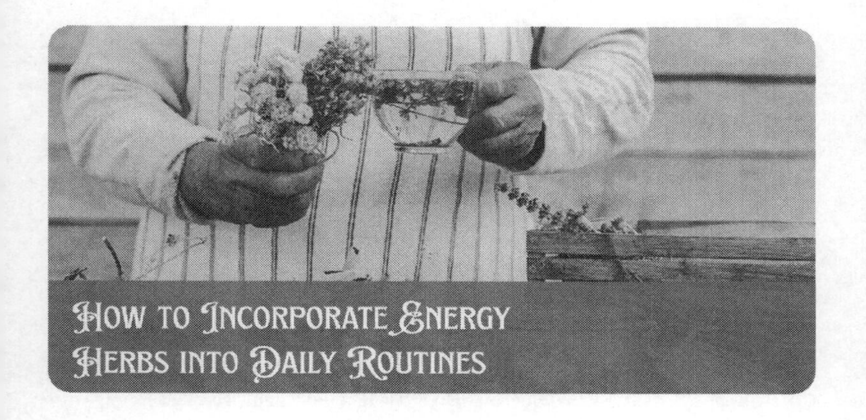

How to Incorporate Energy Herbs into Daily Routines

Incorporating energy-boosting herbs into your daily routine can be both simple and effective. The key is to establish consistent habits that fit seamlessly into your existing routine, ensuring that you benefit from the cumulative effects of the herbs over time. This section offers practical ways to incorporate energy herbs into different parts of your day, from morning rituals to afternoon pick-me-ups.

Morning Rituals

Starting the day with energizing herbs can set a positive tone and provide the stamina needed for a productive morning.

Herbal teas: Brew a cup of yerba mate or ginseng tea as part of your morning ritual. The natural caffeine and adaptogenic properties will energize you without the crash associated with coffee.

Smoothie Booster: Add a teaspoon of maca powder or a dropper of eleuthero tincture to your morning smoothie. This is an easy and delicious way to incorporate adaptogens into your breakfast.

Mindful meditation: Take your morning tincture mindfully. Spend a few moments focusing on your breath and setting an intention for the day as you consume the herbs. This practice can enhance the effectiveness of the herbs and promote mental clarity.

Midday Pick-Me-Ups

The afternoon energy slump is a common experience. Using energy herbs strategically during this time can help maintain focus and stamina.

Herbal infusions: Prepare a midday herbal infusion with Rhodiola and peppermint. This combination can refresh the mind and support sustained energy levels.

Tincture on the Go: Keep a small bottle of eleuthero or rhodiola tincture in your pocket or desk drawer. A few drops in water or tea can provide a quick energy boost when needed.

Eat a healthy snack: Pair your energy herbs with a healthy snack like nuts or fruit to maintain energy. For example, a handful of almonds with a dropper of Maca tincture in a glass of water can work wonders.

Evening Wind-Down

While energy herbs are primarily used to increase stamina, some can also help with evening recovery and stress management.

Post-workout recovery: If you exercise in the evening, consider adding maca or eleuthero tincture to your post-workout smoothie to support muscle recovery and energy restoration.

Adaptogenic Baths: For overall rejuvenation, prepare a warm bath infused with adaptogenic herbs such as ashwagandha or holy basil. While not a direct energy booster, this practice helps your body recover from daily stress and indirectly supports your energy levels.

Incorporating energy herbs into your daily routine can be both enjoyable and practical. Whether through teas, tinctures, or mindful practices, these herbs can help maintain balanced energy and vitality, supporting a more vibrant and fulfilling lifestyle.

CHAPTER 4

Emotional Wellness and Mental Clarity Teas

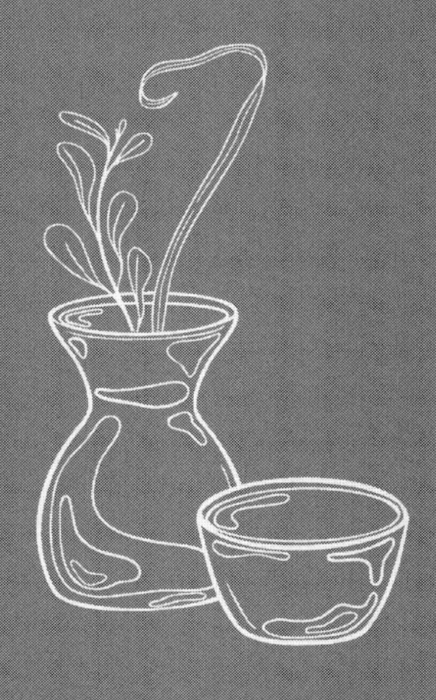

Mental and emotional well-being are fundamental aspects of overall health, yet they are often overlooked in the hustle and bustle of daily life. Herbal teas can be a powerful and soothing way to promote emotional well-being, uplift the spirit, and improve mental clarity. In this chapter, we explore a number of herbal blends that offer natural support for mood, motivation, and cognitive function.

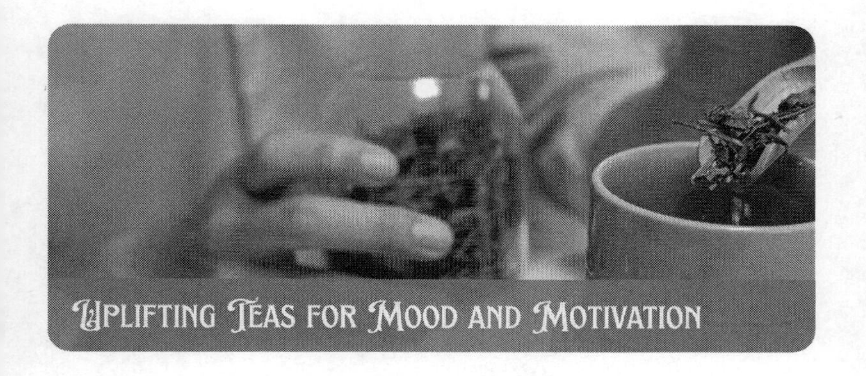

Uplifting Teas for Mood and Motivation

Life's challenges can sometimes make it difficult to stay positive and motivated. Fortunately, certain herbs have been used for centuries to lift your mood and promote a sense of well-being. Blending these herbs into teas is a gentle and enjoyable way to lift your spirits.

St. John's Wort (*Hypericum perforatum*)

St. John's wort is perhaps one of the most well-known herbs for mood support. Traditionally used to relieve symptoms of mild depression and anxiety, it is thought to work by increasing levels of serotonin, dopamine, and norepinephrine - neurotransmitters that play a role in mood regulation.

Primary Benefits:

- ***Mood Stabilization:*** St. John's Wort is effective in reducing feelings of sadness and promoting emotional balance.
- ***Nervous System Support:*** It helps calm an overactive nervous system, making it useful for those experiencing emotional stress.

Precautions: St. John's wort may interact with certain medications, including antidepressants and birth control pills. Always consult a healthcare professional before use.

How to Prepare St. John's Wort Tea:

- ***Ingredients:***1 teaspoon dried St. John's wort flowers, hot water, honey (optional).

- ***Method:*** Steep the dried flowers in hot water for 5 to 10 minutes. Strain and sweeten with honey if desired. Drink 1 to 2 cups daily for best results.

Lemon Balm (*Melissa officinalis*)

Lemon Balm is a fragrant herb known for its calming yet uplifting effects. It is commonly used to reduce anxiety and promote a sense of peace, making it a valuable addition to any mood-boosting tea blend.

Primary Benefits:

- ***Anxiety Relief:*** Lemon Balm helps to calm the mind and lift the spirit, making it useful for those who experience nervousness or mood swings.
- ***Digestive Aid:*** It also supports digestion, which can be impacted by stress and emotional upheaval.

Blending Tip: Lemon Balm pairs well with other uplifting herbs, such as lavender and chamomile.

How to Prepare Lemon Balm Tea:

- ***Ingredients:***1 tablespoon dried lemon balm leaves, hot water, a slice of fresh lemon (optional).
- ***Method:*** Steep the leaves in hot water for 5 to 7 minutes. Add a slice of lemon for extra zest and enjoy.

Holy Basil (Tulsi) (*Ocimum sanctum*)

Holy Basil, also known as Tulsi, is revered in Ayurvedic medicine for its adaptogenic properties, which help the body adapt to stress. It is known to elevate mood, improve mental clarity, and increase resilience to physical and emotional stress.

Primary Benefits:

- *Stress Reduction:* Tulsi helps reduce cortisol levels, alleviating the physical and emotional effects of stress.
- ***Mental Clarity:*** It increases focus and supports a balanced mood, making it ideal for times when motivation is low.

How to Prepare Holy Basil Tea:

- ***Ingredients:***1 teaspoon dried basil leaves, 1/2 teaspoon dried peppermint (optional), hot water.

- *Method:* Steep the holy basil leaves in hot water for 5 to 10 minutes. Add peppermint for a refreshing twist and enjoy throughout the day.

Rose (*Rosa spp.*)

Rose petals are not only visually beautiful, but also have a calming and uplifting effect on the mind. Rose tea is often used to relieve emotional distress and to promote self-love and compassion.

Primary Benefits:

- ***Emotional Balance:*** Rose petals help release pent-up emotions and reduce feelings of sadness or frustration.
- ***Heart Health:*** The calming effect of rose tea extends to the physical heart, promoting cardiovascular health.

How to Prepare Rose Tea:

- ***Ingredients:***1 tablespoon dried rose petals, 1 teaspoon honey (optional), hot water.
- ***Method:*** Steep rose petals in hot water for 5 to 7 minutes. Sweeten with honey and enjoy as a gentle reminder to care for your emotional well-being.

Uplifting Tea Blends for Everyday Motivation

Creating blends that combine these herbs can enhance their effectiveness and provide a balanced approach to emotional wellness.

Sample Recipe for a Mood-Boosting Tea:

- 1 teaspoon St. John's Wort
- 1 tablespoon Lemon Balm
- 1 teaspoon dried Rose petals
- Steep in hot water for 5 to 10 minutes, strain, and enjoy warm.

Whether you're starting your day or need an afternoon pick-me-up, these uplifting teas can support a brighter mood and renewed motivation. The next section explores calming tinctures for those moments when you need to relax and find your center.

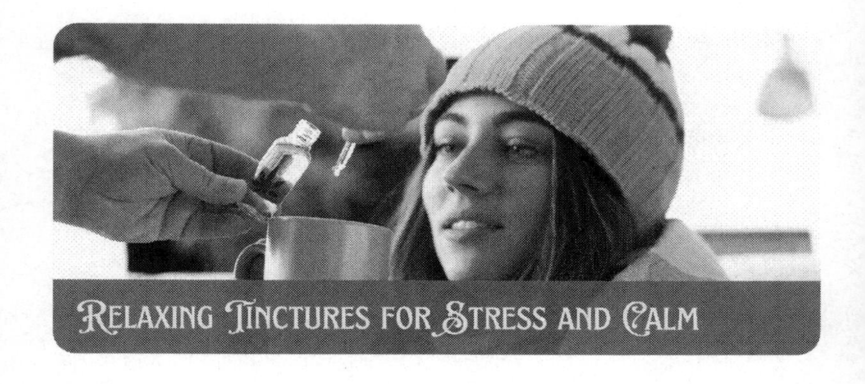

Relaxing Tinctures for Stress and Calm

In a world filled with constant demands and stress, finding a natural way to calm the mind and body is invaluable. Relaxation tinctures made from carefully selected herbs offer an effective and convenient way to relieve stress and restore balance. These alcohol-free extracts are easy to use, making them a practical option for those looking to manage stress in a holistic way.

Skullcap (*Scutellaria lateriflora*)

Skullcap is a powerful nervine herb known for its ability to calm an overactive mind and relax the nervous system. It is often used to treat anxiety, restlessness, and sleep disturbances caused by stress. The active ingredients in Skullcap, such as flavonoids and baicalin, work to reduce nervous tension and promote a sense of calm.

Primary Benefits:

Nervous System Support: Skullcap is highly effective in reducing stress-related tension and promoting relaxation without causing drowsiness.

Anxiety Relief: It helps alleviate feelings of worry and supports emotional well-being, making it a go-to herb for managing daily stress.

Preparation: To make a skullcap tincture, use dried skullcap herb and glycerin or vinegar as a solvent. Fill a sterilized jar one-third full with dried skullcap, cover with the solvent of your choice, and macerate for 4 to 6 weeks. Strain and store in a dark glass bottle.

Lavender (*Lavandula angustifolia*)

Lavender is widely appreciated for its soothing and calming

properties. It is particularly useful for those who experience anxiety, tension headaches, or insomnia. The aromatic compounds in lavender work to calm the mind and relax the body, creating a sense of calm and peace.

Primary Benefits:

Anxiety Reduction: Lavender's calming scent and gentle sedative properties make it an excellent herb for reducing anxiety and promoting relaxation.

Sleep Aid: For those who have trouble sleeping due to stress, lavender can help relax the body and prepare the mind for a restful slumber.

Preparation: Combine dried lavender flowers with glycerin or apple cider vinegar in a sterilized jar. Allow the mixture to macerate for 4 to 6 weeks, shaking the jar daily. Strain the tincture and store in a cool, dark place.

California Poppy (*Eschscholzia californica*)

California Poppy is a mild sedative and anxiolytic herb often used to calm the mind and promote restful sleep. Unlike stronger sedatives, it does not leave you feeling groggy the next day, making it suitable for daytime use in small doses.

Primary Benefits:

Mild Sedative Effects: California Poppy helps reduce anxiety and promotes deep relaxation, making it ideal for use at night or during times of high stress.

Pain Relief: It also has mild analgesic properties, which can be beneficial for tension headaches or muscle aches related to stress.

Preparation: Use dried California poppy herb to make a non-alcoholic tincture. Follow the same method of maceration and storage, and be sure to label the tincture with the date and herb used.

Relaxation tinctures are a versatile and powerful tool for managing stress naturally. They can be taken directly under the tongue or added to a cup of soothing herbal tea for an enhanced effect.

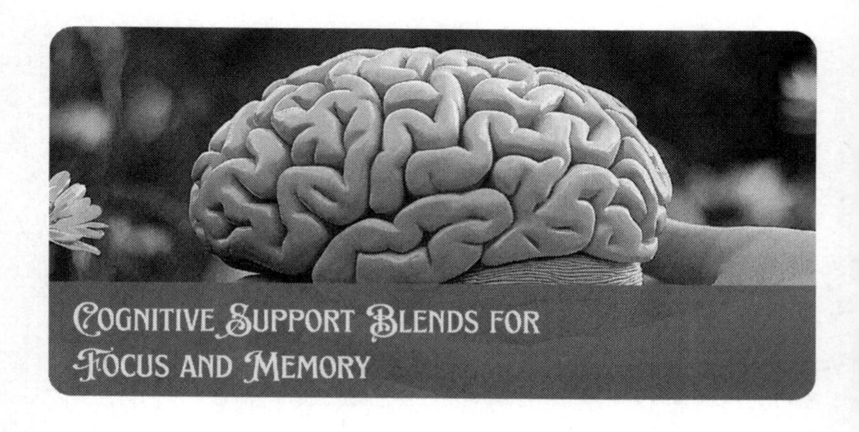

Cognitive Support Blends for Focus and Memory

In today's fast-paced world, mental clarity and focus are more important than ever. Herbal blends that support cognitive function can help improve memory, sharpen focus, and enhance overall mental performance. By selecting herbs known for their nootropic and adaptogenic properties, you can create teas and tinctures that naturally boost brain power.

Gotu Kola (*Centella asiatica*)

Gotu Kola is a revered herb in traditional medicine, particularly Ayurveda, for its ability to support brain health. It is known to enhance cognitive function, improve memory, and increase concentration. The herb works by increasing blood flow to the brain and supporting neuronal health.

Primary Benefits:

Memory Enhancement: Gotu Kola has neuroprotective properties that improve memory retention and learning abilities.

Focus and Concentration: By increasing blood flow to the brain, it sharpens focus and enhances mental clarity.

How to use: Gotu Kola can be consumed as a tea or made into a tincture. For a tea, steep 1 teaspoon of dried Gotu Kola in hot water for 5 to 10 minutes. For a tincture, follow the same preparation method as above, using either glycerin or vinegar.

Bacopa (*Bacopa monnieri*)

Bacopa, another staple of Ayurvedic medicine, is known for its cognitive-enhancing effects. It is often used to reduce anxiety while improving brain function. Bacopa has been shown to improve synaptic communication, which is critical for learning and memory.

Primary Benefits:

- ***Improved Cognitive Function:*** Bacopa improves mental performance and reduces brain fog, making it a favorite of students and professionals.
- ***Stress Reduction:*** It has adaptogenic properties that help balance stress hormones, indirectly benefiting brain health.

How to use: Bacopa can be taken as a tea or tincture. A bacopa tea can be made by steeping 1 teaspoon of dried bacopa leaves in hot water. Alternatively, you can make a tincture using dried bacopa leaves and your favorite non-alcoholic solvent.

Rosemary (*Rosmarinus officinalis*)

Rosemary is not only a flavorful culinary herb but also a potent cognitive enhancer. The aromatic compounds in rosemary have been shown to improve memory and concentration. It is particularly effective when inhaled as well as ingested.

Primary Benefits:

Memory Support: Rosemary improves recall and learning by enhancing cerebral blood flow.

Mental Clarity: The invigorating aroma of rosemary can reduce mental fatigue and promote alertness.

How to use: Rosemary tea can be made by steeping a few sprigs of fresh rosemary or 1 teaspoon of dried rosemary in hot water. You can also make a tincture using dried rosemary, following the standard method of preparation.

These cognitive support blends offer a natural way to improve focus and memory without the need for synthetic stimulants. Whether through teas, tinctures, or even aromatherapy, these herbs provide a comprehensive approach to maintaining mental sharpness and clarity.

CHAPTER 5

Seasonal Teas for Immune and Digestive Health

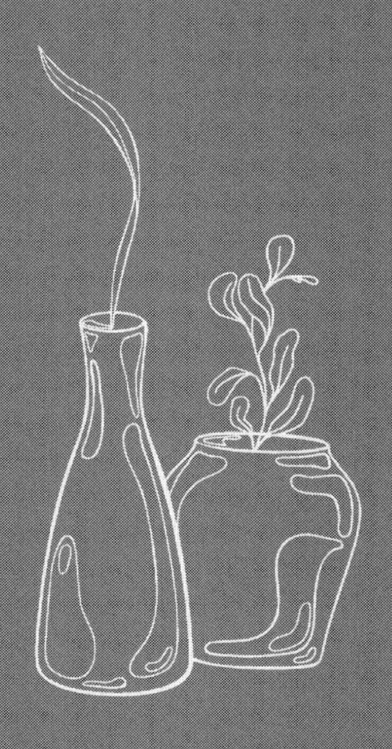

Maintaining a robust immune system and a healthy digestive tract throughout the year requires a seasonal approach. As our bodies adjust to different environmental and dietary factors, seasonal herbal teas can provide targeted support to boost immunity and promote optimal digestion. This chapter explores how to harness the power of herbs through tailored tea blends for each season.

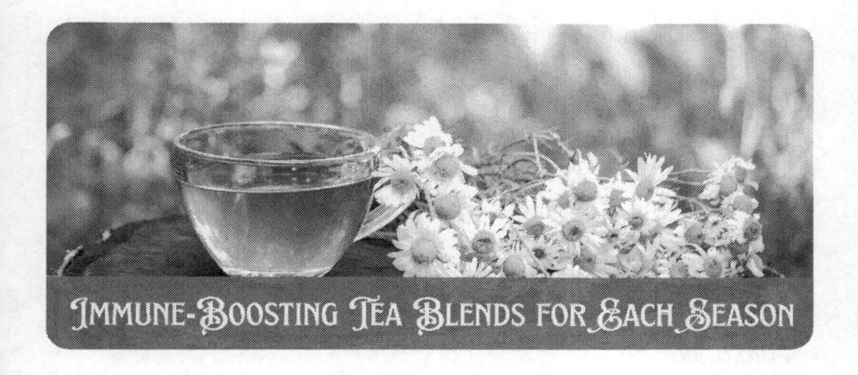

Immune-Boosting Tea Blends for Each Season

Seasonal changes can challenge the immune system, so it is important to adjust our diet and wellness practices accordingly. Incorporating specific herbal teas tailored to each season can provide targeted support to strengthen immunity throughout the year.

Spring: Nettle and Dandelion Tea

Spring is a time of renewal, and supporting the body's natural detoxification processes can improve immune function. Nettle (*Urtica dioica*) is rich in vitamins A and C, which are essential for immune health. Dandelion (*Taraxacum officinale*) supports liver function and aids in the elimination of toxins. Combining these herbs creates a tea that revitalizes and prepares the body for the warmer months.

Preparation: Steep 1 teaspoon each of dried nettle and dandelion leaves in 8 ounces of boiling water for 10 minutes. Strain and enjoy up to twice daily.

Summer: Hibiscus and Elderflower Tea

In summer, hydration and antioxidant support are essential. Hibiscus (*Hibiscus sabdariffa*) is rich in vitamin C and antioxidants, supporting immune health and providing a refreshing taste. Elderflower (*Sambucus nigra*) is traditionally used to support respiratory health and strengthen the immune system. This combination provides a cooling and immune-supporting beverage.

Preparation: Steep 1 teaspoon each of dried hibiscus petals and elderflowers in 8 ounces of boiling water for 5-7 minutes. Strain and serve hot or iced.

Autumn: Astragalus and Cinnamon Tea

As the weather cools, strengthening the immune system becomes a priority. Astragalus (*Astragalus membranaceus*) is an adaptogen known for its immune-boosting properties. Cinnamon (*Cinnamomum verum*) adds warmth and has antimicrobial properties. Together, they create a tea that prepares the body for the challenges of the colder months.

Preparation: Simmer 1 tablespoon of dried astragalus root in 16 ounces of water for 20 minutes. Add a cinnamon stick during the last 5 minutes. Strain and drink up to twice daily.

Winter: Rosehip and Ginger Tea

Winter brings increased susceptibility to colds and flu. Rosehips (*Rosa canina*) are high in vitamin C, which supports immune function. Ginger (*Zingiber officinale*) provides warmth and has antiviral properties. This tea offers both immune support and comfort during the cold season.

Preparation: Steep 1 teaspoon of dried rose hips and a few slices of fresh ginger in 8 ounces of boiling water for 10 minutes. Strain and enjoy up to three times daily.

By tailoring herbal tea consumption to seasonal needs, we can provide our bodies with the specific support they need to maintain robust immune health throughout the year.

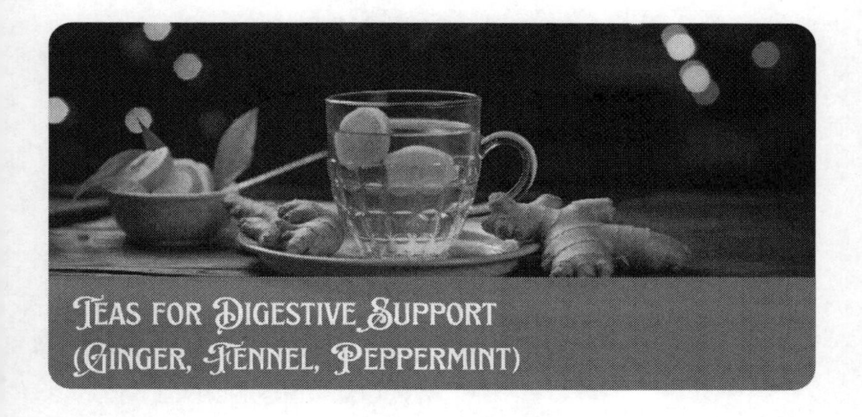

Teas for Digestive Support (Ginger, Fennel, Peppermint)

Digestive health is fundamental to overall well-being, as the gut plays an important role in nutrient absorption, immune function, and mental health. Herbal teas offer a gentle yet effective way to support digestive processes, soothe an upset stomach, and relieve bloating or indigestion. Key herbs such as ginger, fennel, and peppermint are widely recognized for their digestive benefits.

Ginger (*Zingiber officinale*)

Ginger is a powerful digestive aid known for its ability to relieve nausea, reduce bloating, and stimulate digestion. Its anti-inflammatory properties make it ideal for soothing an irritated gut, while its warming effect helps break down food more efficiently.

Primary Benefits:

Relieves Nausea: Ginger is particularly effective against nausea and vomiting, making it a staple for motion sickness and pregnancy-induced morning sickness.

Reduces Bloating: By stimulating the production of digestive enzymes, ginger helps break down food and relieves gas and bloating.

Anti-Inflammatory: Ginger's active compounds, such as gingerol, reduce inflammation in the gut and promote digestive comfort.

To make ginger tea: Slice a thumb-sized piece of fresh ginger and steep in hot water for 10 minutes. Add honey or a slice of lemon for extra flavor. Drink before or after meals to aid digestion.

Fennel (*Foeniculum vulgare*)

Fennel seeds are a traditional remedy for digestive disorders, especially for gas and bloating. The seeds contain essential oils that have carminative properties, helping to relax the muscles in the digestive tract and reduce gas formation.

Primary Benefits:

Relieves Bloating and Gas: Fennel helps expel gas trapped in the digestive tract, making it ideal for those who experience frequent bloating.

Promotes Digestion: The seeds stimulate the secretion of digestive enzymes, aiding in the breakdown of food.

Anti-Spasmodic: Fennel relaxes the smooth muscles of the intestines, reducing cramps and discomfort.

How to make fennel tea: Crush 1 teaspoon of fennel seeds and steep in hot water for 5 to 7 minutes. Strain and drink warm, especially after meals.

Peppermint (*Mentha piperita*)

Peppermint is known for its cooling and soothing effects on the digestive system. It relaxes the muscles of the gastrointestinal tract, making it effective for treating irritable bowel syndrome (IBS) and general digestive discomfort.

Key Benefits:

Reduces Indigestion: Peppermint tea may relieve symptoms of indigestion, such as bloating and gas, by calming stomach muscles and improving bile flow.

Relieves Irritable Bowel Syndrome: The menthol in peppermint has a relaxing effect on the muscles of the bowel, reducing spasms and discomfort associated with Irritable Bowel Syndrome.

Freshens Breath: Beyond digestion, peppermint leaves a refreshing aftertaste and helps combat bad breath.

To make peppermint tea: Steep 1 tablespoon of dried peppermint leaves in hot water for 5 to 10 minutes. Drink after meals to aid digestion and reduce bloating.

By incorporating these digestive teas into your daily routine, you can support a healthy gut and enjoy relief from common digestive complaints.

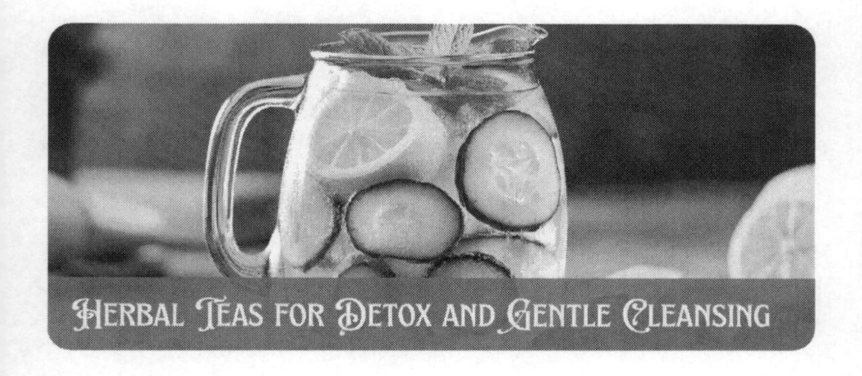

Herbal Teas for Detox and Gentle Cleansing

Detoxification is a natural process the body uses to eliminate toxins and waste products. However, in today's world of pollutants and processed foods, the body can benefit from extra support. Herbal teas formulated for gentle cleansing can support the liver, kidneys, and lymphatic system, promoting overall well-being without harsh effects.

Dandelion Root (*Taraxacum officinale*)

Dandelion root is a well-known liver tonic that stimulates bile production, aiding in the digestion and elimination of fats. It also acts as a gentle diuretic, helping to flush excess water and toxins from the body.

Key Benefits:

Liver Support: Dandelion root helps detoxify the liver, promoting the efficient breakdown and elimination of waste products.

Diuretic: It gently increases urine production, aiding in the removal of toxins through the kidneys.

Nutrient Rich: Dandelion root is packed with vitamins and minerals, providing nutrition while supporting detoxification.

How to make dandelion root tea: Simmer 1 tablespoon of dried dandelion root in 8 ounces of water for 10 to 15 minutes. Strain and drink once daily for a gentle cleansing.

Burdock Root (*Arctium lappa*)

Burdock root is a powerful blood purifier that has been used for centuries to support liver function and remove toxins from the bloodstream. It also promotes healthy skin and supports the lymphatic system.

Primary Benefits:

Blood Purification: Burdock root helps remove impurities from the blood, making it beneficial for skin conditions such as acne or eczema.

Lymphatic Support: It stimulates lymphatic drainage, helping the body to eliminate waste products.

Anti-Inflammatory Properties: Burdock root reduces inflammation in the liver and digestive tract.

How to make burdock root tea: Simmer 1 teaspoon of dried burdock root in 2 cups of water for 15 minutes. Strain and drink up to twice a week as part of a detoxification program.

Red Clover (*Trifolium pratense*)

Red Clover is a gentle detoxifying herb that supports the lymphatic system and helps cleanse the blood. It is known for its ability to promote skin health and provide relief from chronic inflammatory conditions.

Key Benefits:

Lymphatic System Support: Red Clover helps move lymphatic fluid and eliminate toxins from the body.

Skin Health: By purifying the blood, it reduces skin problems such as rashes or acne.

Hormonal Balance: Red clover also contains phytoestrogens, which can help balance hormones during detoxification.

How to make red clover tea: Steep 1 to 2 teaspoons of dried red clover flowers in hot water for 10 minutes. Drink daily as part of a gentle detox program.

Incorporating these detox teas into your wellness routine is a natural and gentle way to support your body's cleansing processes and promote overall health and vitality.

CHAPTER 6

Teas and Tinctures for Women's Health

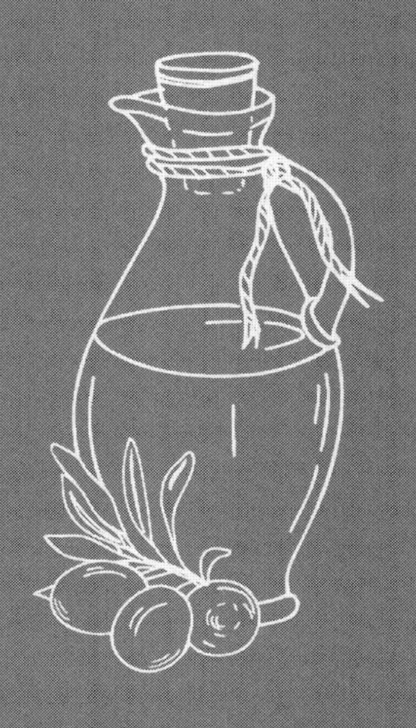

Women's health encompasses a range of unique needs and concerns, from hormonal balance to reproductive health and prenatal care. Herbal teas and tinctures offer a gentle yet effective approach to addressing these areas, supporting the body's natural processes, and promoting overall well-being. This chapter explores how specific herbs can be used to make teas and tinctures to support hormonal support, menstrual health, and pregnancy care.

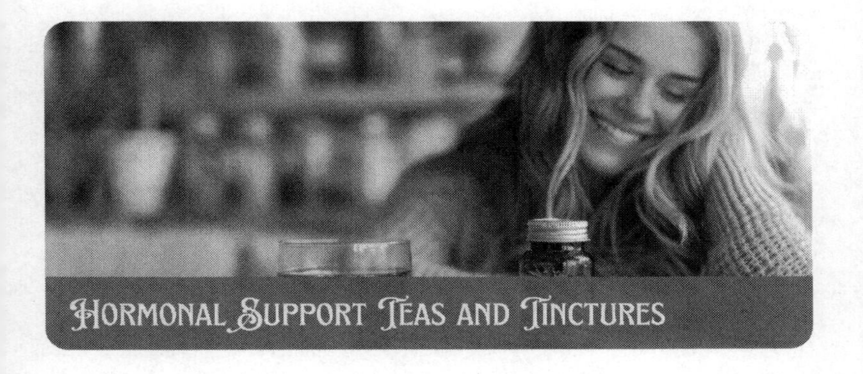

Hormonal Support Teas and Tinctures

Hormonal imbalances can affect many aspects of a woman's health, from mood and energy levels to reproductive function and skin health. Herbal remedies that help balance hormones can be invaluable in promoting physical and emotional stability. This section focuses on herbal teas and tinctures designed to support the endocrine system and naturally regulate hormones.

Chaste Tree Berry (*Vitex agnus-castus*)

Chaste Tree Berry, also known as Vitex, is one of the most widely used herbs for balancing female hormones. It acts on the pituitary gland, helping to regulate the production of progesterone and other hormones. Vitex is especially beneficial for conditions like premenstrual syndrome (PMS), irregular periods, and hormonal acne.

Primary Benefits:

Regulates menstrual cycle: Vitex helps normalize the menstrual cycle, making it useful for women who experience irregular periods.

Reduces PMS Symptoms: It may reduce common PMS symptoms such as breast tenderness, bloating, and mood swings by balancing hormones.

Supports Fertility: By promoting a healthy balance of estrogen and progesterone, Vitex may improve fertility.

How to use: Vitex can be taken as a tea or a tincture. To make a tincture, soak dried vitex berries in glycerin or vinegar for 4 to 6 weeks. Take 1 to 2 teaspoons daily for optimal hormonal support.

Red Raspberry Leaf (*Rubus idaeus*)

Red Raspberry Leaf is known as the "woman's herb" for its extensive reproductive health benefits. It is rich in vitamins and minerals, including iron, calcium, and magnesium, which help strengthen the uterus and support overall hormonal health.

Key Benefits:

Uterine Tonic: Red Raspberry Leaf tones the uterus, making it beneficial for menstrual health and fertility.

Nutrient Rich: The vitamins and minerals in the leaf support hormone production and overall reproductive well-being.

Relieves Menstrual Cramps: It may reduce the severity of menstrual cramps and promote a smoother menstrual flow.

Suggested Use: To make a tea, steep 1 to 2 teaspoons of dried red raspberry leaf in hot water for 10 minutes. Drink daily as a general tonic for women's health.

Dong Quai (*Angelica sinensis*)

Dong Quai, often called "female ginseng," is a traditional Chinese herb used to support hormonal balance and improve blood flow to the reproductive organs. It is particularly effective for menopausal symptoms and menstrual irregularities.

Key Benefits:

Balances Hormones: Dong Quai may help relieve symptoms of menopause, such as hot flashes and mood swings, by regulating estrogen levels.

Improves Circulation: It increases blood flow to the pelvic area, which may help with menstrual cramps and other reproductive problems.

Relieves PMS Symptoms: The anti-inflammatory properties of dong quai make it useful for reducing the pain and discomfort associated with PMS.

How to use: Dong Quai is most commonly used in tincture form. Combine dried dong quai root with glycerin or apple cider vinegar and steep for 4 to 6 weeks. Take 1 to 2 teaspoons daily, but consult a health care professional if you are pregnant or taking blood-thinning medications.

Holy Basil (Tulsi) (*Ocimum sanctum*)

Holy Basil, or Tulsi, is an adaptogenic herb that helps the body adapt to stress and balance cortisol levels. Since stress is a major contributor to hormonal imbalance, Tulsi is an excellent herb for overall hormonal support.

Primary Benefits:

Reduces Stress: Tulsi helps lower cortisol levels, promoting emotional and hormonal balance.

Supports Metabolism: By improving metabolic function, it helps maintain a healthy weight, which is important for hormonal health.

Anti-Inflammatory: Tulsi has anti-inflammatory and antioxidant properties that protect the endocrine system.

Usage: Brew a cup of tulsi tea by steeping 1 teaspoon of dried holy basil leaves in hot water for 5 to 10 minutes. Drink daily, especially during periods of high stress.

Hormonal balance is critical to a woman's well-being, and these teas and tinctures provide a natural, effective way to support the body. In the following sections, we'll explore herbal remedies specifically designed for menstrual and reproductive health.

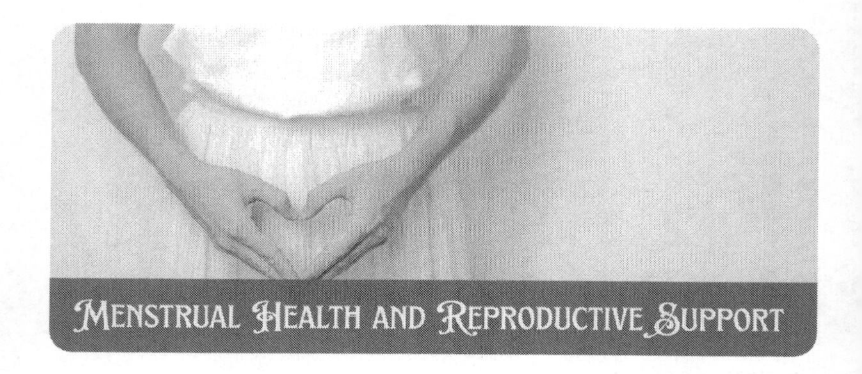

Menstrual Health and Reproductive Support

Menstrual health is an important aspect of women's well-being, and many women experience a variety of discomforts associated with their menstrual cycles, such as cramps, heavy bleeding, and mood swings. Herbal remedies have long been used to relieve these symptoms and promote reproductive health. Herbs that support menstruation work by regulating hormones, reducing inflammation, and nourishing the reproductive system.

Cramp Bark
(*Viburnum opulus*)

Cramp Bark is a powerful herb traditionally used to relieve menstrual cramps and muscle spasms. It works by relaxing the smooth muscles of the uterus, which can significantly reduce the intensity of menstrual pain.

Primary Benefits:

Relieves Menstrual Cramps: Cramp Bark's antispasmodic properties help ease uterine contractions, providing relief from severe cramps.

Reduces Muscle Tension: It may also help relieve lower back pain and other muscle aches associated with menstruation.

Supports Healthy Blood Flow: By promoting circulation, Cramp Bark ensures a smoother menstrual flow.

How to use: Cramp bark is most commonly consumed as a tea or tincture. To make a tea, steep 1 to 2 teaspoons of dried cramp bark in hot water for 10 to 15 minutes. Drink up to three times a day during your menstrual cycle.

Yarrow (*Achillea millefolium*)

Yarrow is a versatile herb known for its ability to regulate menstrual flow and tone the uterus. It can help women who experience heavy menstrual flow and irregular periods by promoting balance and stability in the reproductive system.

Primary Benefits:

Balances menstrual flow: Yarrow helps reduce excessive bleeding and may also encourage a delayed onset of menstruation, promoting regularity.

Anti-Inflammatory: Its anti-inflammatory properties may relieve pelvic congestion and discomfort.

Uterine Tonic: Yarrow strengthens the uterine muscles, making it useful for women who experience weakness in their reproductive organs.

Usage: Yarrow tea can be made by steeping 1 teaspoon of dried yarrow flowers in hot water for 10 minutes. Drink up to twice daily, especially during heavy periods.

Shatavari (*Asparagus racemosus*)

Shatavari is a well-known herb in Ayurvedic medicine that supports the female reproductive system. It is used to increase fertility, balance hormones, and relieve menopausal symptoms. Shatavari nourishes and rejuvenates the reproductive organs, making it an essential herb for women at various stages of life.

Primary Benefits:

Balances Hormones: Shatavari helps regulate estrogen levels, making it beneficial for both menstrual and menopausal symptoms.

Enhances Fertility: It supports egg health and strengthens the uterine lining, increasing the chances of a healthy pregnancy.

Relieves PMS Symptoms: Shatavari's calming and nourishing properties may reduce mood swings, bloating, and irritability.

How to use: Shatavari is most effective as a tincture or powdered supplement. Add 1/2 to 1 teaspoon of shatavari powder to warm milk or water and drink daily for ongoing support.

Motherwort (*Leonurus cardiaca*)

Feverfew is a calming herb known for its ability to relieve menstrual cramps, reduce anxiety, and regulate irregular periods. It has a grounding effect, making it an excellent choice for women who experience emotional upheaval during their menstrual cycle.

Key Benefits:

Relieves Menstrual Cramps: Feverfew's antispasmodic properties soothe the uterus and reduce pain.

Regulates Irregular Periods: It promotes a regular menstrual cycle, especially in women who have irregular periods due to hormonal imbalances.

Calms the Nervous System: Feverfew helps reduce anxiety and stress, which can be exacerbated by hormonal fluctuations.

Directions: Take 1 to 2 teaspoons of feverfew tincture up to twice daily during your menstrual cycle. Avoid using feverfew if you are pregnant as it may stimulate uterine contractions.

These herbal remedies offer a natural approach to menstrual health and reproductive support, helping women experience a more balanced and comfortable cycle.

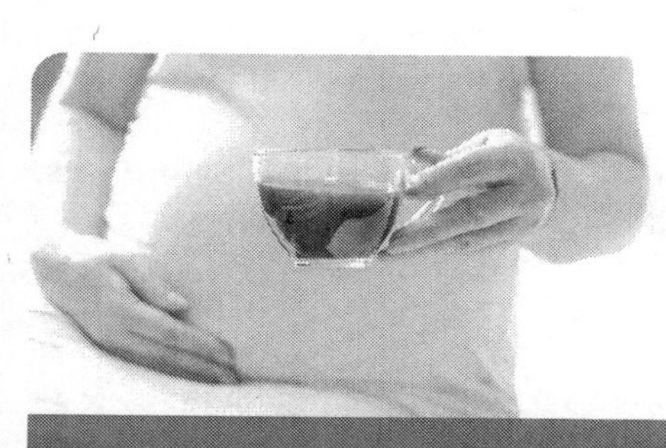

Prenatal and Postnatal Herbal Support

Pregnancy and the postpartum period are times of immense change, both physically and emotionally. Herbal teas and tinctures can provide gentle yet effective support for women during these times, nourishing the body and aiding in recovery. It's important to choose herbs that are safe for both mother and baby, focusing on nutrition, relaxation, and uterine health.

Red Raspberry Leaf (*Rubus idaeus*)

Red Raspberry Leaf is one of the most revered herbs for pregnancy and postpartum care. It is rich in vitamins and minerals, including iron, calcium, and magnesium, and is known to strengthen the uterus, making labor and delivery more efficient.

Key Benefits:

Uterine Tonic: Red Raspberry Leaf tones the uterine muscles, preparing the body for labor and promoting postpartum recovery.

Nutrient Rich: It provides essential nutrients that support the health of both mother and baby.

Lactation Support: Red Raspberry Leaf may also help increase milk supply for breastfeeding mothers.

How to use: Prepare a nourishing tea by steeping 1 to 2 teaspoons of dried Red Raspberry Leaf in hot water for 10 minutes. Drink daily during pregnancy and postpartum for continued support.

Nettle (*Urtica dioica*)

Nettle is a nutrient powerhouse, providing vitamins A, C, and K, as well as iron and calcium. It supports the overall health of pregnant women and helps prevent anemia, a common problem during and after pregnancy.

Key Benefits:

Iron-Rich: Nettle's high iron content helps prevent and treat anemia, ensuring that the mother has adequate energy levels.

Bone and Joint Health: The calcium in nettle supports the skeletal health of both mother and baby.

Postpartum Recovery: Nettle helps replenish nutrients lost during childbirth and supports lactation.

Directions: Steep 1 tablespoon of dried nettle leaves in hot water for 10 minutes. Drink up to 2 cups daily, especially during the third trimester and postpartum period.

Oatstraw (*Avena sativa*)

Oatstraw is a calming and nourishing herb that supports the nervous system and is a rich source of vitamins and minerals. It is especially helpful in reducing stress and promoting relaxation during pregnancy and the postpartum period.

Key Benefits:

Calms the nervous system: Oatstraw helps reduce anxiety and promotes restful sleep, which can be challenging during pregnancy.

Rich in Nutrients: It provides magnesium, calcium, and B vitamins to support the body's overall strength and resilience.

Supports Lactation: Oatstraw may also help increase milk supply in breastfeeding mothers.

How to use: Make an oatstraw infusion by steeping 1 tablespoon of dried oatstraw in a quart of hot water for several hours. Strain and drink throughout the day for continuous nutrition.

Fenugreek (*Trigonella foenum-graecum*)

Fenugreek seeds are commonly used to increase milk supply in breastfeeding mothers. They contain phytoestrogens that stimulate milk production and help maintain an adequate supply.

Key Benefits:

Increases Milk Supply: Fenugreek is one of the most effective galactagogues for promoting lactation.

Aids Digestion: It also supports digestive health, which can be beneficial during the postpartum period.

Anti-Inflammatory Properties: Fenugreek helps reduce inflammation, aiding in recovery after childbirth.

How to use: Make a fenugreek tea by boiling 1 teaspoon of crushed seeds in water for 10 minutes. Strain and drink once a day, but consult a healthcare provider to make sure it's appropriate for your needs.

Prenatal and postnatal herbal support can make a significant difference in a woman's overall well-being by providing nourishment, calming the mind, and aiding in recovery. As with any herbal remedy, it's important to consult with a healthcare provider to ensure safety and appropriateness for your individual situation.

CHAPTER 7

Creating Custom Teas and Tinctures for Family Use

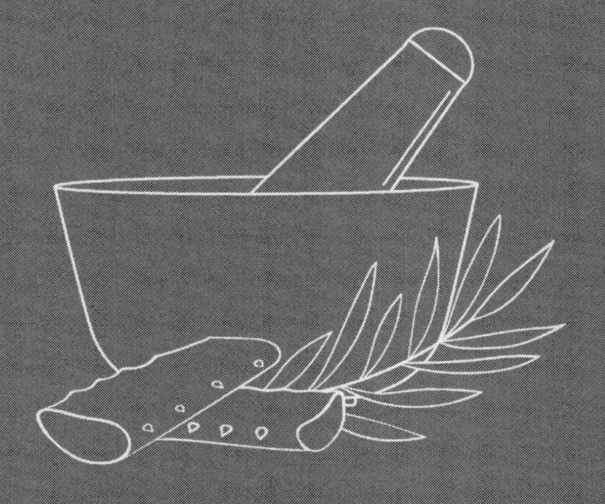

When it comes to caring for the whole family, herbal teas and tinctures offer a versatile and effective approach. With the right blends, you can address the unique needs of each family member, from infants to the elderly. By creating custom formulations, you can tailor herbal remedies to promote health and well-being for everyone. This chapter will guide you through creating safe and nutritious formulas for children, elderly family members, and the entire household.

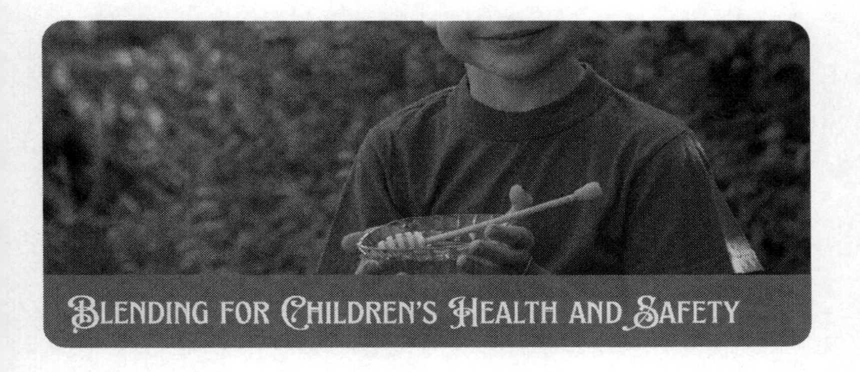

Blending for Children's Health and Safety

Children need special care when it comes to herbal remedies. Their developing bodies are sensitive, and it's important to use herbs that are both gentle and effective. Blends for children focus on boosting immunity, soothing common ailments such as coughs and colds, and calming hyperactivity or anxiety.

Chamomile (*Matricaria chamomilla*)

Chamomile is one of the safest and most effective herbs for children. Known for its calming properties, it can be used to soothe upset stomachs, relieve teething pain, and promote restful sleep. Chamomile also supports the immune system, making it an excellent choice for general wellness.

Key Benefits:

Calming: Chamomile helps relax an anxious or overactive child, making it useful at bedtime or in stressful situations.

Digestive Support: It relieves digestive upsets such as gas and colic.

Teething Relief: Chamomile tea can be applied topically to relieve the pain of teething.

How to use: Make a gentle tea by steeping 1 teaspoon of dried chamomile flowers in hot water for 5 minutes. Strain and allow to cool before serving to a child. For infants, use a clean cloth to apply the cooled tea to the gums.

Lemon Balm (*Melissa officinalis*)

Lemon balm is a gentle herb that is perfect for children who are feeling anxious or have trouble sleeping. It has a pleasant, lemony flavor and can help calm upset stomachs, making it a favorite of parents and children alike.

Key Benefits:

Reduces Anxiety: Lemon balm calms the nervous system and promotes emotional balance in children.

Digestive Aid: It relieves indigestion and upset stomach caused by stress or diet.

Immune Support: The herb has mild antiviral properties that may help ward off the common cold.

Usage: Steep 1 teaspoon of dried lemon balm in hot water for 5 minutes. Allow the tea to cool before serving to children. It can also be mixed with chamomile for a stronger calming effect.

Elderflower (*Sambucus nigra*)

Elderflower is a mild herb that supports the immune system and is especially helpful during cold and flu season. It can reduce fever and relieve respiratory discomfort, making it a valuable addition to children's wellness routines.

Key Benefits:

Immune Support: Elderflower helps the body fight off infections and may shorten the duration of a cold.

Respiratory: It relieves congestion and soothes irritated airways.

Anti-Inflammatory: The herb reduces inflammation, aiding in faster recovery.

How to use: Make a light tea by steeping 1 teaspoon of dried elderflower in hot water for 5 minutes. Cool and serve as needed, or mix with honey for added soothing properties (for children over one year of age).

Creating safe herbal formulas for children requires careful consideration, but the right herbs can make a significant difference in promoting health and well-being. Always consult a pediatrician before introducing any new herbs, especially for very young children or those with medical conditions.

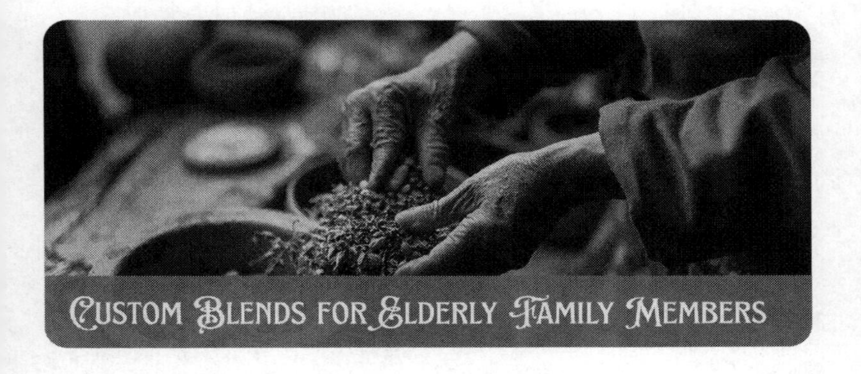

Custom Blends for Elderly Family Members

As family members age, their bodies require specific, gentle, yet effective herbal support to maintain health and vitality. The elderly often face a variety of age-related issues, such as joint pain, weakened cardiovascular systems, cognitive decline, and digestive problems. Customized herbal blends can be a wonderful way to address these concerns holistically, ensuring that aging family members feel nourished and supported.

One of the primary concerns for older adults is joint and muscle health. Chronic inflammation can lead to conditions such as arthritis, causing daily discomfort and limiting mobility. A warm, soothing tea blend can help alleviate some of this pain while promoting flexibility and reducing inflammation. An effective blend for this purpose includes turmeric and ginger, both known for their powerful anti-inflammatory properties. Turmeric contains curcumin, a compound with powerful antioxidant and anti-inflammatory properties that can be beneficial for reducing joint pain.

When combined with ginger, which also has warming, anti-inflammatory properties, the two herbs create a synergistic effect that relieves discomfort. To make a potent tea, slice fresh ginger and combine it with ground turmeric in hot water and steep for about ten minutes. This tea can be sipped throughout the day for ongoing relief.

In addition to pain management, cardiovascular health is a critical consideration for the elderly. The heart and circulatory system can weaken over time, increasing the risk of conditions such as high blood pressure and heart disease. Hawthorn Berry is one of the best herbs to support heart health, as it has been used for centuries to strengthen the heart and improve circulation.

Hawthorn Berry tea is rich in flavonoids, which have antioxidant and vasodilator effects, helping to relax blood vessels and promote healthy blood pressure levels. To make a heart-healthy tea, boil dried hawthorn berries in water for about fifteen minutes.

Drinking this regularly can help strengthen the heart and support overall cardiovascular function. Paired with cinnamon, which is not only delicious but also has blood sugar regulating properties, this blend becomes even more beneficial for an aging heart.

Digestive health is another key area where the elderly may need extra support. Over time, the digestive system can become sluggish, leading to problems such as bloating, constipation, and indigestion. Herbs such as fennel and peppermint can be particularly helpful in promoting digestive well-being. Fennel acts as a natural carminative, helping to calm the gastrointestinal tract and relieve gas. It also has mild laxative properties that can help relieve constipation. Peppermint, on the other hand, calms the digestive muscles, making it useful for treating symptoms of irritable bowel syndrome and indigestion. Together, these herbs can be steeped to make a refreshing and effective digestive aid, perfect for drinking after meals.

For cognitive health, a blend that includes rosemary and ginkgo biloba can be incredibly supportive. Rosemary has long been associated with improved memory and mental clarity. Its aromatic compounds may help improve concentration and cognitive function. Ginkgo biloba, a well-known nootropic herb, increases blood flow to the brain, which may be beneficial in preventing age-related cognitive decline.

Combining these two herbs in a daily tea can create a brain-boosting tonic that keeps the mind sharp and engaged. Simply steep dried rosemary leaves and ginkgo biloba in hot water and encourage older family members to drink this blend regularly as part of their wellness routine.

Finally, it is important to consider the emotional well-being of older adults. Aging can be associated with feelings of isolation, anxiety, or depression, and calming, mood-lifting herbs can make a significant difference. Lavender and lemon balm are two excellent choices for promoting relaxation and reducing anxiety. Lavender tea is known for its ability to calm the nervous system and relieve stress, while lemon balm gently lifts the mood and may even improve sleep quality.

A soothing evening tea made with these herbs can help older family members wind down at the end of the day and promote restful and restorative sleep.

Creating custom herbal blends to meet the unique needs of elderly family members is a heartfelt way to care for them. These teas can provide not only physical relief, but also a sense of comfort and nurturing that helps older adults feel cared for and valued.

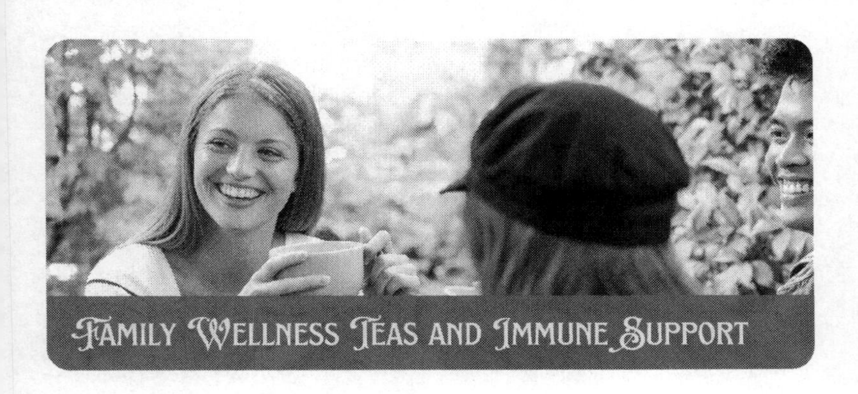

Family Wellness Teas and Immune Support

The well-being of an entire family often depends on the collective health of each member. From the youngest to the oldest, keeping everyone healthy is a top priority, especially during cold and flu season. Family wellness teas, designed to boost the immune system and provide a soothing experience, can play an integral role in maintaining overall health. These blends are meant to be shared, creating a sense of unity and warmth within the household.

A basic family immune support tea includes echinacea and elderberry. Echinacea is known for its ability to stimulate the immune system, making it more efficient at fighting off infections. It is especially effective when taken at the first sign of illness, helping to reduce the duration and severity of colds and flu. Elderberry, with its antiviral and antioxidant properties, complements Echinacea perfectly.

Rich in vitamins A, B, and C, elderberry boosts immune function and is especially effective against respiratory viruses. To make a family-friendly tea, steep echinacea and elderberries in hot water and add honey for a touch of sweetness that children will enjoy. This tea can be enjoyed warm or iced, making it a versatile addition to any wellness routine.

For families with young children, it is important to create a gentle and soothing tea that provides immune support without being too strong. Chamomile and lemon balm are an excellent combination for this purpose. Chamomile is a calming herb that can reduce anxiety and promote sleep, while also having mild antimicrobial properties.

Lemon Balm adds a pleasant lemony flavor and helps calm the nervous system, making it perfect for fussy children who need to relax. This blend can be served in the evening to help promote a restful sleep and ensure that little ones are well rested and ready to face the day. Parents can also enjoy this tea to unwind after a long day, creating a shared moment of peace and relaxation.

During the colder months, a warming and immune-boosting tea of astragalus and cinnamon can help keep the family healthy. Astragalus is an adaptogen that supports the immune system over time, making it a great herb for daily use. It helps the body adapt to stress and increases overall resilience.

Cinnamon, with its warming and antimicrobial properties, adds flavor and aids digestion, which is essential for maintaining a healthy immune system. A pot of astragalus and cinnamon tea simmering on the stove fills the home with a soothing aroma, inviting everyone to gather and share in the benefits of this nourishing brew.

Family wellness also extends to digestive health, which plays a critical role in overall immunity. A tea blend of ginger and licorice root can support both digestion and the immune system. Ginger warms the body and aids digestion, while licorice root soothes the digestive tract and has antiviral properties. This blend can be especially helpful after a heavy meal or during times of digestive discomfort. The naturally sweet flavor of licorice root makes this tea appealing to children, while adults will appreciate its soothing effects.

For a versatile, all-purpose wellness tea, consider a blend that includes peppermint, rose hips, and hibiscus. Peppermint provides a refreshing taste and aids digestion, while rose hips are packed with vitamin C, an important nutrient for immune support. Hibiscus adds a tart, fruity flavor and is rich in antioxidants, making this tea a beautiful and healthful option. The bright red color of this tea is visually appealing, encouraging even the pickiest family members to take a sip.

These family wellness teas create an opportunity for everyone to come together and focus on their health in a natural and enjoyable way. Whether it's a warm cup shared around the kitchen table on a chilly day or a refreshing iced tea sipped in the summer sun, these herbal blends provide more than just physical nourishment-they foster a sense of togetherness and shared well-being that strengthens the family bond.

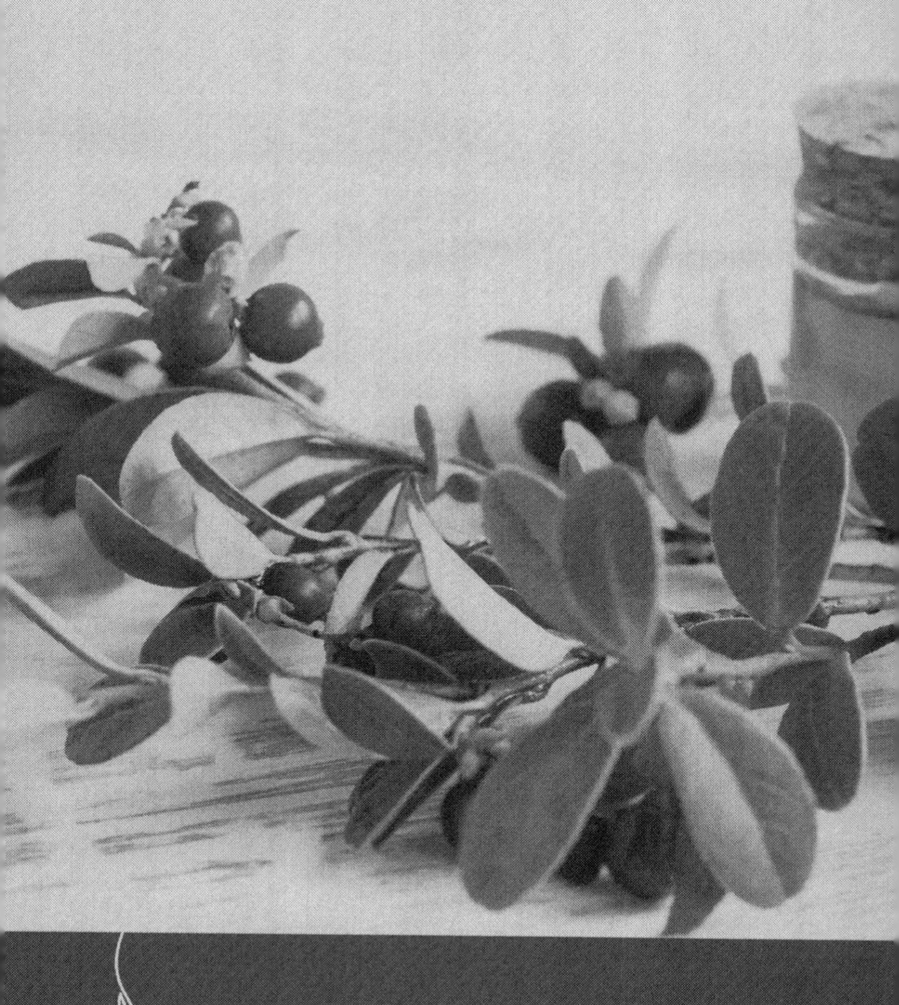

BOOK 03

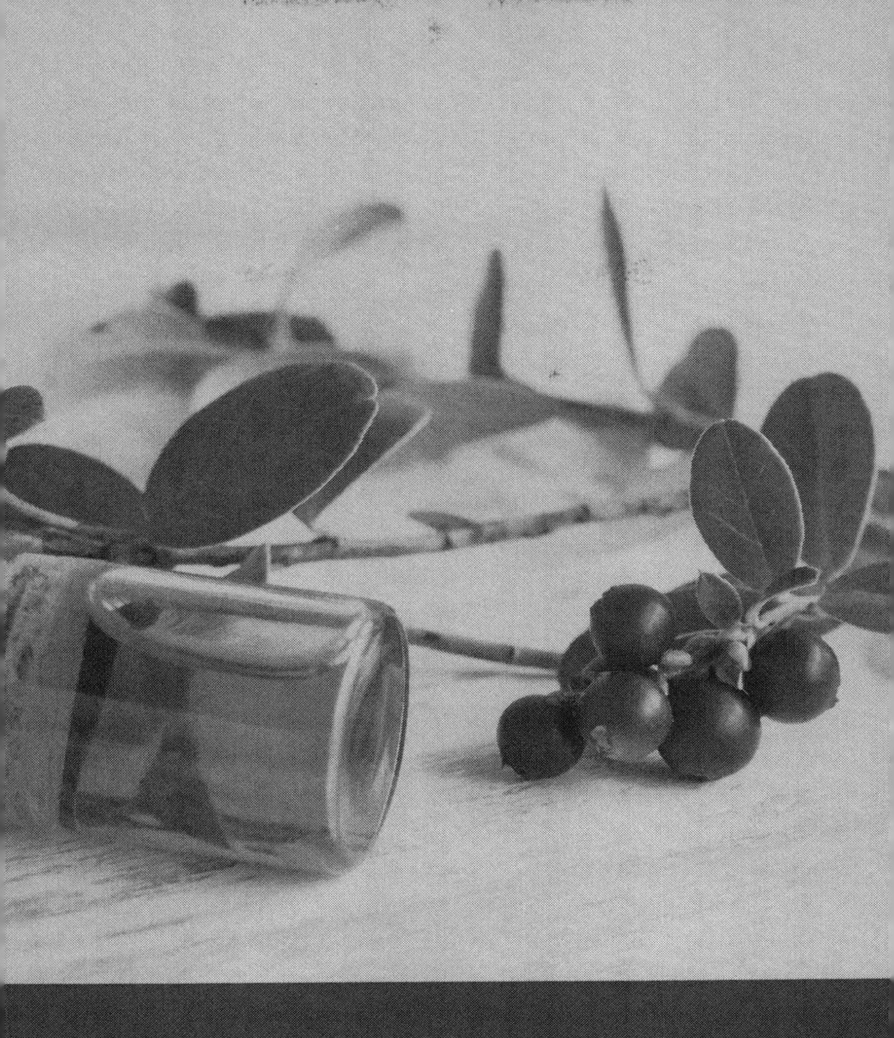

Essential Oils and Balms for Healing and Self-Care

Essential oils have been used for thousands of years in various cultures for their therapeutic properties and ability to support physical, emotional and spiritual well-being. These potent plant extracts are a versatile and effective addition to any self-care routine, offering benefits that range from promoting relaxation and reducing stress to soothing skin conditions and relieving pain. This book will guide you through the essential knowledge needed to use oils safely and effectively, create your own healing balms, and establish a holistic, nature-based self-care practice.

CHAPTER 1

Getting Started with Essential Oils

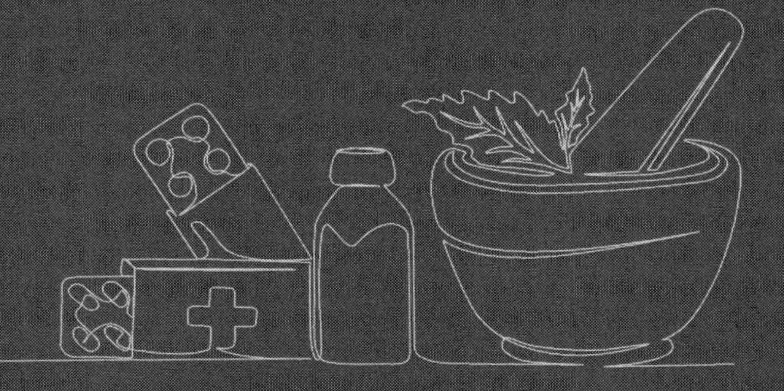

Embarking on a journey with essential oils opens up a world of natural healing possibilities. However, given the potency and complexity of these plant extracts, understanding the basics is critical to ensuring safe and effective use. This chapter covers everything you need to know to get started, from selecting high-quality oils to understanding safety practices and proper dilution.

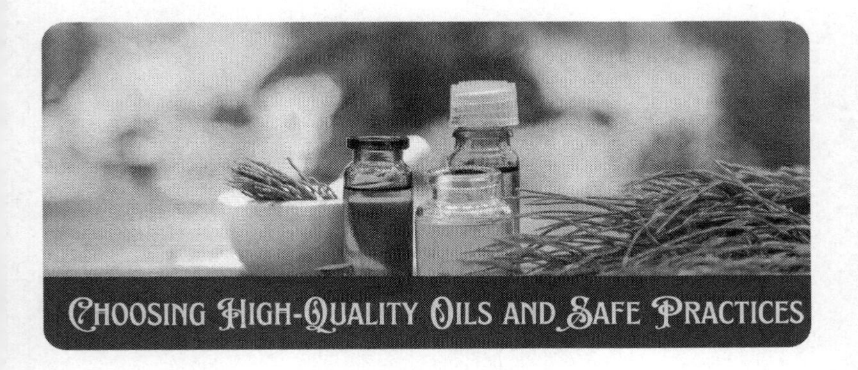

Choosing High-Quality Oils and Safe Practices

The quality of essential oils is paramount, as the purity and potency of the oil directly affects its effectiveness and safety. Not all essential oils on the market are created equal. Many are diluted, adulterated, or made from inferior plant material, which can compromise their therapeutic properties and even pose risks. When choosing essential oils, it is important to invest in reputable brands that prioritize quality and transparency.

High-quality essential oils should be 100% pure and come from carefully sourced plant material. Look for oils that are labeled with the botanical name of the plant (e.g., *Lavandula angustifolia* for true lavender), the country of origin, and the method of extraction. Companies that provide third-party test results, such as GC/MS (gas chromatography/mass spectrometry) reports, are more likely to offer authentic products. These reports confirm the chemical composition of the oil and ensure that there are no contaminants or synthetic additives.

Organic certification is another factor to consider, especially for oils derived from crops that are heavily sprayed with pesticides. Organic oils come from plants grown without synthetic fertilizers or pesticides, making them a safer and more environmentally friendly option. It is also important to understand the harvesting practices and sustainability of the oil. Essential oils such as sandalwood and frankincense come from trees that can be overharvested, so it is important to choose brands that support ethical and sustainable sourcing.

Once you have chosen your oils, it is important to understand how to use them safely. Essential oils are highly concentrated and should never be applied directly to the skin without dilution. They must always be mixed with a carrier oil, such as coconut, jojoba, or almond oil, to prevent skin irritation or sensitization. Even inhaling essential oils requires some caution; while diffusing them is generally safe, it is important to limit exposure time and ensure proper ventilation, especially when using oils around children, pregnant women, or pets.

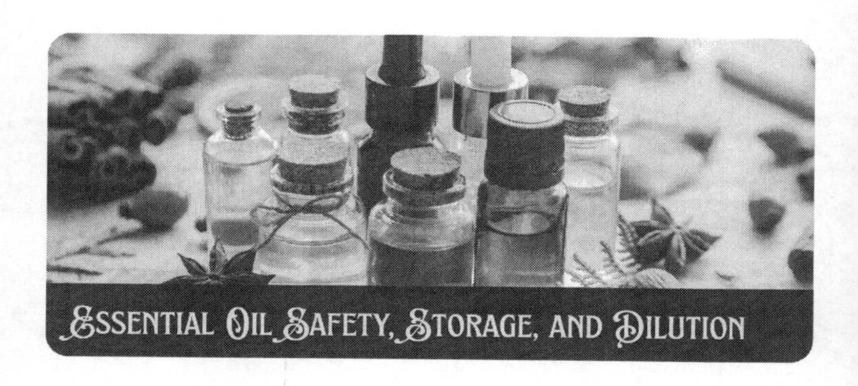

Essential Oil Safety, Storage, and Dilution

Safety is the cornerstone of effective essential oil use. Due to their concentrated nature, these oils can cause adverse reactions if not used properly. Understanding dilution ratios, proper storage, and safety guidelines ensures that you can enjoy the benefits of essential oils while minimizing the risks.

Dilution is essential when using oils topically. A common guideline is to dilute essential oils to 1-3% for adults, depending on the oil and purpose of use. This translates to approximately 6-18 drops of essential oil per ounce (30 ml) of carrier oil. For more sensitive populations, such as children, the elderly, or those with compromised immune systems, a lower dilution of 0.5-1% is recommended. Always patch test before using a new oil to ensure there are no allergic reactions.

Certain oils are phototoxic, meaning they can increase the skin's sensitivity to sunlight and cause burns or skin discoloration when exposed to UV rays. Citrus oils such as bergamot, lemon and lime are notorious for this effect and should be used with caution. When applying phototoxic oils topically, avoid direct sun exposure for at least 12-24 hours or use in areas covered by clothing.

Proper storage of essential oils is also critical to maintaining their potency and shelf life. Essential oils should be stored in dark glass bottles away from heat, light, and air. Exposure to these elements can cause the oils to oxidize and lose their therapeutic properties. Keeping oils in a cool, dark place, such as a cabinet or refrigerator, will help preserve their quality. Also, make sure the caps are tightly closed to prevent evaporation and oxidation.

Some essential oils have a shorter shelf life than others. Citrus oils, for example, tend to oxidize more quickly and should be used within one to two years. On the other hand, oils like patchouli and sandalwood can improve with age, becoming richer and more complex over time. Keeping track of purchase dates and labeling your bottles can help you monitor the freshness of your oils.

Special precautions must be taken when using essential oils for children or during pregnancy. Certain oils, such as peppermint and eucalyptus, are too strong for young children and may cause difficulty breathing. Oils such as clary sage and rosemary should be avoided during pregnancy as they may stimulate the uterus. Always consult a qualified aromatherapist or healthcare provider when using essential oils in these sensitive situations.

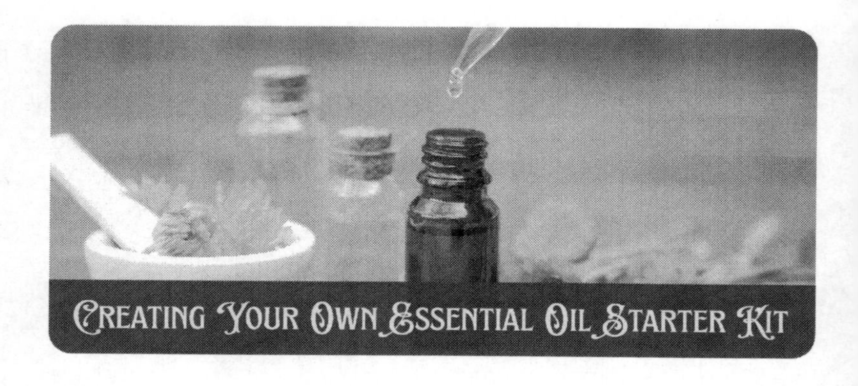

Creating Your Own Essential Oil Starter Kit

Beginning your essential oil journey can be overwhelming with the wide variety of oils available. Building a basic kit of versatile, high-quality essential oils is a convenient way to get started and explore the many benefits they offer. A well-rounded starter kit typically includes oils that can address common concerns such as stress, minor aches and pains, skin irritations, and respiratory problems.

One of the most important oils to have in your kit is lavender. Known for its calming and soothing properties, lavender can be used to promote relaxation, improve sleep, and soothe minor skin irritations such as burns and insect bites. It is gentle enough for children and can be diffused, added to bath water, or diluted for topical application.

Another essential oil is tea tree, known for its antimicrobial and antifungal properties. Tea tree oil is a powerful remedy for skin infections, acne, and minor wounds, making it an essential addition to any natural first aid kit.

Peppermint is another versatile oil known for its cooling and invigorating properties. It can be used to relieve headaches, soothe muscle tension, and improve focus and energy. When diluted and applied to the abdomen, peppermint oil is also effective in relieving digestive discomfort and bloating. Eucalyptus is a respiratory powerhouse, helping to clear congestion and support lung health. It is excellent for use in steam inhalations or air diffusion during cold and flu season.

Frankincense, often called the "King of Oils," offers a wide range of benefits, from supporting the immune system to promoting healthy skin and reducing inflammation. It is grounding and can be used in meditation practices as well as blended with carrier oils for skin care. Finally, lemon oil is a bright and uplifting addition to any kit. It can purify the air, increase energy, and can be used as a natural cleaner when diluted in water.

Once you have your essential oils, assembling a starter kit involves organizing your collection for easy access. Use a sturdy wooden or metal box to store your oils and label each bottle clearly. You may also want to include a small selection of carrier oils, glass roller bottles for making your own blends, and pipettes for accurate measurements. Keeping a notebook or journal to record your experiences and favorite recipes can also be helpful as you become more familiar with your essential oils.

Starting with a curated collection of essential oils sets the stage for a holistic approach to self-care and healing. As you gain confidence and experience, you can expand your kit to include more specialized oils, experiment with different blends, and discover the full potential of these natural remedies.

CHAPTER 2

DIY Balms and Salves for Skin and Muscle Relief

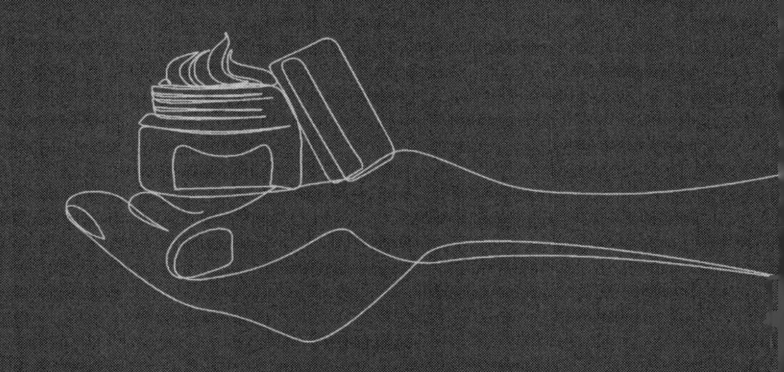

Balms and ointments are some of the most accessible and effective ways to harness the healing power of herbs and essential oils. They are easy to make at home and provide a natural solution to common skin and muscle problems.

Unlike creams or lotions, which are water-based, balms and salves are oil-based, making them more concentrated and effective for deep hydration and targeted relief. This chapter will guide you through creating your own herbal balms and salves for a variety of uses, from soothing irritated skin to relieving sore muscles.

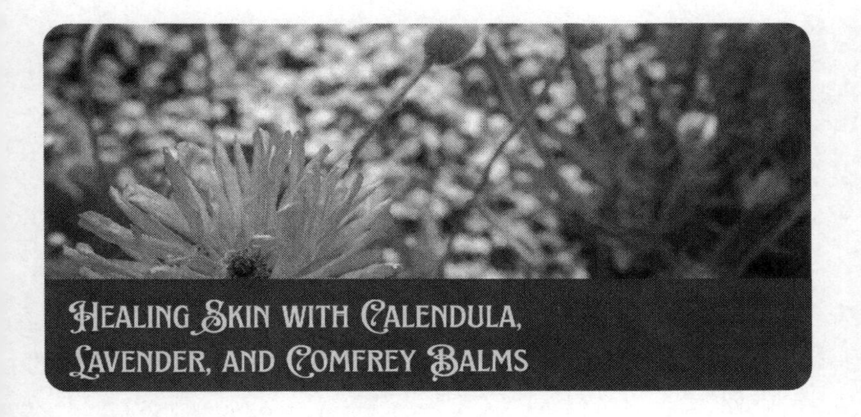

Healing Skin with Calendula, Lavender, and Comfrey Balms

The skin is the body's largest organ and often the first line of defense against environmental stressors. So it's no surprise that it needs extra care and attention, especially when it's dealing with wounds, dryness, or irritation.

Calendula, lavender and comfrey are three herbs known for their exceptional skin-healing properties, making them ideal for creating a nourishing and soothing balm.

Calendula, also known as marigold, is renowned for its anti-inflammatory and skin-regenerating properties. Gentle enough for sensitive skin, it can be used to treat minor cuts, rashes, and eczema. The bright orange petals of the calendula flower are infused into carrier oils to extract their healing compounds, resulting in a vibrant golden oil that forms the base of a restorative skin balm. In addition to reducing redness and swelling, calendula stimulates the production of collagen, which is essential for wound healing.

Lavender, another essential ingredient in skin balms, provides a calming and antiseptic effect. Known for its soothing scent, lavender is perfect for reducing inflammation and speeding healing of burns, insect bites, and dry patches.

Lavender essential oil contains linalool, a compound that soothes irritated skin and provides a natural defense against infection. When combined with calendula, lavender enhances the overall effectiveness of the balm, providing both antibacterial protection and a soothing, aromatic experience.

Comfrey, often called "knitbone," is a powerful herb used to speed the healing of wounds, bruises, and sprains. It contains allantoin, a substance that promotes cell regeneration and helps repair damaged tissue. Comfrey is particularly effective for treating minor abrasions and deeply moisturizing dry or chapped skin. It should be used with caution, however, as it is potent and best suited for short-term use. The addition of comfrey to a skin balm provides a robust formula for treating everything from scraped knees to rough, weathered hands.

To make a healing skin balm, you would first infuse a blend of dried marigold, lavender, and comfrey in a carrier oil such as olive or jojoba oil. This infusion can be left to steep for several weeks or gently heated to speed up the process. Once the oil is ready, it is mixed with beeswax to solidify the balm and make it easy to apply. The final product can be stored in small jars and used as needed to nourish and protect the skin.

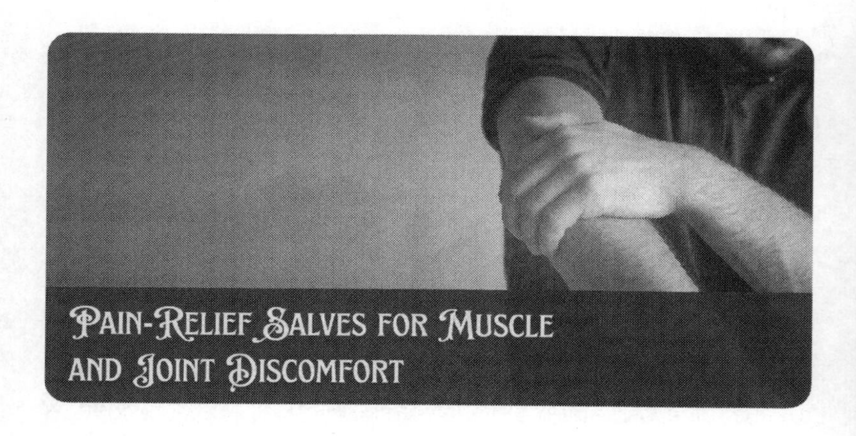

Pain-Relief Salves for Muscle and Joint Discomfort

Whether it's from strenuous exercise, chronic conditions like arthritis, or simply the physical demands of everyday life, muscle and joint pain are common ailments that many people experience. Herbal ointments with pain-relieving and anti-inflammatory ingredients can provide natural relief by penetrating deep into the tissues to relieve soreness and promote healing. The key to an effective pain-relieving salve is to use a combination of warming and cooling herbs to attack discomfort from multiple angles.

Arnica is one of the best-known herbs for reducing inflammation and relieving pain. It is often used by athletes to relieve sore muscles, bruises, and joint pain. The active compounds in arnica, known as sesquiterpene lactones, help reduce swelling and improve blood flow to the affected area. Arnica-infused oil forms the base of many pain-relieving ointments and provides immediate relief when massaged into sore muscles or stiff joints.

In addition to arnica, cayenne pepper is an excellent pain reliever. It contains capsaicin, a compound that temporarily reduces the sensation of pain by blocking the neurotransmitters responsible for sending pain signals to the brain. The warming effect of cayenne increases blood flow to the area, helping to relax muscles and loosen joints. However, cayenne should be used in moderation, as it can cause irritation if the concentration is too high. The combination of arnica and cayenne in an ointment creates a powerful remedy for pain that provides both immediate and long-lasting relief.

Wintergreen essential oil, which contains natural methyl salicylate, is another powerful pain reliever. It mimics the effects of aspirin and can be used to reduce inflammation and ease muscle and joint discomfort. When added to an ointment, wintergreen provides a cooling sensation that soothes sore areas, making it an excellent complement to the warming properties of cayenne. This combination of warming and cooling provides a balanced approach to pain relief.

To make a pain-relieving salve, start by infusing arnica and cayenne in a high-quality carrier oil, such as olive or avocado oil. When the infusion is ready, melt beeswax into the oil and add a few drops of wintergreen essential oil. The resulting ointment can be applied to sore muscles and joints, providing relief from everything from post-exercise soreness to arthritis pain.

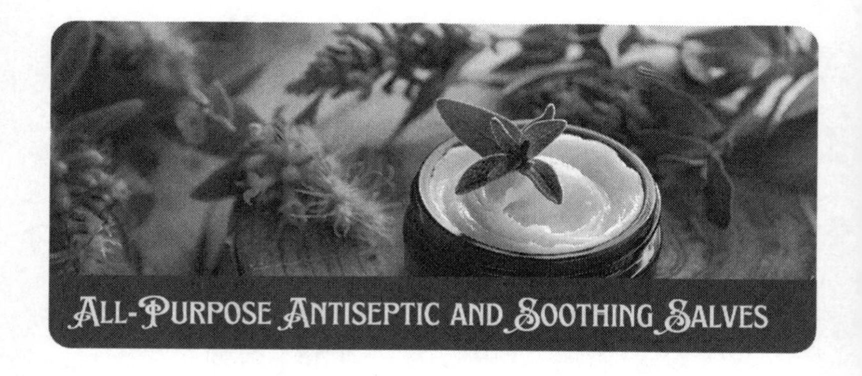

All-Purpose Antiseptic and Soothing Salves

An all-purpose antiseptic and soothing ointment is a must in any natural first aid kit. These versatile salves can be used to treat minor cuts, scrapes, insect bites, and skin irritations, providing both antibacterial protection and soothing relief. The combination of antiseptic and healing herbs helps keep the skin free of infection while promoting quick recovery.

Tea Tree Oil is a staple in antiseptic salves due to its powerful antibacterial, antifungal and antiviral properties. It is effective against a wide range of pathogens, making it ideal for treating wounds and preventing infections. Despite its strength, tea tree oil is gentle enough to be used on most skin types and can help reduce redness and swelling. When combined with other soothing ingredients, tea tree oil provides comprehensive protection and speeds the healing process.

Plantain, a common herb found in backyards and gardens, is another excellent addition to an all-purpose salve. It has natural drawing properties that make it effective for pulling out splinters, soothing bee stings, and relieving the itchiness of insect bites. Plantain is also anti-inflammatory and can help soothe skin irritations, making it a valuable herb for general skin care. Infusing plantain leaves in a carrier oil and blending it with tea tree oil creates a powerful base for an antiseptic salve.

Beeswax plays a critical role in the formulation of these salves, creating a protective barrier over the skin that locks in moisture and prevents dirt and bacteria from entering the wound. The waxy consistency also ensures that the salve stays in place, providing long-lasting relief and healing. The addition of soothing herbs such as marigold and chamomile enhances the balm's soothing effect, reducing pain and inflammation while supporting the skin's natural healing process.

To make an all-purpose antiseptic ointment, combine tea tree oil, plantain infused oil, and a blend of soothing herbs in a base of melted beeswax. Once the salve has cooled and solidified, it can be stored in a small jar and used whenever minor injuries or skin irritations occur. This versatile balm is a natural, effective way to keep skin healthy and protected, whether it's a skinned knee or an annoying insect bite.

Making your own DIY balms and salves empowers you to take control of your health and care for your skin and muscles naturally. With the right combination of herbs and essential oils, you can create targeted remedies that provide lasting relief and promote overall wellness. These recipes are not only effective, but also offer a personal touch, allowing you to customize each balm to meet the needs of your family.

CHAPTER 3

Essential Oil Blends for Mood and Relaxation

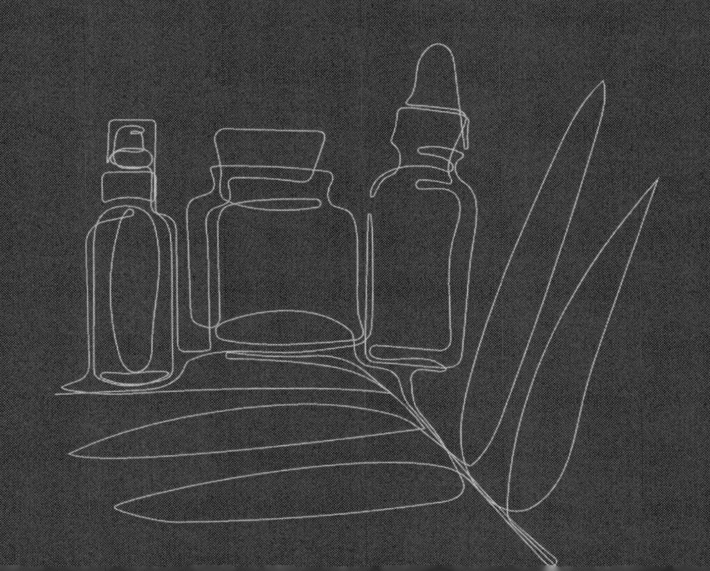

Essential oils are potent plant extracts that have long been used for their therapeutic and emotional benefits. They can have a profound impact on our mental and emotional well-being, providing support for a variety of needs, from reducing anxiety and promoting restful sleep to increasing focus and enhancing meditation practices. This chapter focuses on creating essential oil blends that can help you manage stress, find clarity, and establish a sense of inner peace.

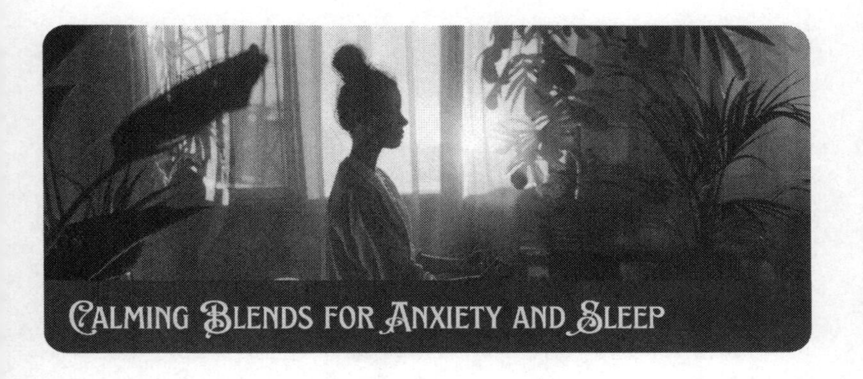

Calming Blends for Anxiety and Sleep

In today's fast-paced world, anxiety and sleep disturbances are increasingly common. The soothing aroma of certain essential oils can help calm the mind, reduce stress, and prepare the body for deep, restorative sleep. Creating calming blends involves selecting oils known for their ability to relax the nervous system, promote feelings of safety, and induce tranquillity.

One of the most effective oils for managing anxiety and promoting relaxation is bergamot. Bergamot has a citrusy yet slightly floral scent that lifts the spirit while calming frayed nerves. It works well with grounding oils such as cedarwood, which has a warm, woody aroma that brings a sense of stability and comfort. Together, bergamot and cedarwood create a blend that gently relieves feelings of tension and creates an environment conducive to relaxation.

For those who struggle with sleep, vetiver is a grounding oil that helps calm a restless mind. Vetiver's deep, earthy scent can be incredibly soothing, especially when combined with Roman Chamomile, a floral oil known for its calming properties. Roman chamomile has a mild, apple-like aroma that soothes the senses and promotes deep, restful sleep. Blended with vetiver, it is a powerful remedy for insomnia and overactive thoughts.

Another classic combination for anxiety and sleep is ylang-ylang and clary sage. Ylang-ylang is known for its sweet, floral scent, which helps lower blood pressure and promotes a sense of joy and relaxation. Clary Sage, on the other hand, has a slightly musky, herbal scent that is effective in relieving tension and balancing hormones. Together, these oils can be diffused in the evening to create a calming atmosphere, or diluted in a carrier oil for a soothing massage before bed.

To use these calming blends, consider adding a few drops to a diffuser, creating a pillow spray, or mixing them with a carrier oil for a calming massage. You can also create a bedtime ritual by applying a diluted blend to your pulse points, allowing the relaxing aromas to signal your body that it's time to unwind.

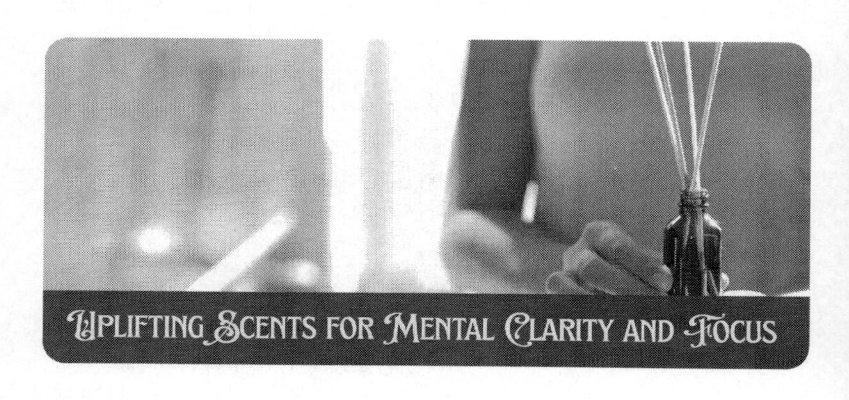

Uplifting Scents for Mental Clarity and Focus

Mental clarity and focus are essential for productivity and overall well-being. Essential oils can act as natural stimulants, helping to clear mental fog, improve concentration and enhance cognitive function. When creating blends for focus and mental clarity, it's important to choose oils that invigorate the mind while providing a balanced sense of energy.

Peppermint is a popular choice for increasing focus and sharpening the senses. Its cool, minty aroma stimulates the brain, increases alertness, and promotes a sense of freshness. The combination is especially effective when used with rosemary, another cognitive enhancing oil. Rosemary has a strong, herbal scent that has been shown to improve memory retention and mental performance. Together, peppermint and rosemary create an energizing blend that is perfect for diffusing in a work or study area.

Citrus oils like lemon and grapefruit are also fantastic for uplifting the mind. Lemon has a bright, zesty scent that invigorates the senses and improves concentration, while grapefruit adds a slightly sweeter, more refreshing note. These oils are mood elevators, lifting spirits and promoting a positive mental state. A blend of lemon, grapefruit and a touch of basil can create a powerful aroma that inspires creativity and keeps you focused on the task at hand.

For those who experience mid-afternoon slumps, eucalyptus and frankincense can be a revitalizing combination. Eucalyptus has a fresh, camphor-like scent that opens the airways and increases oxygen flow to the brain, improving concentration and alertness. Frankincense, known for its grounding and balancing properties, helps maintain a steady flow of energy without causing overstimulation. Together, these oils create a harmonious blend that provides clarity and a sense of purpose.

Using these uplifting blends is easy. You can add them to a diffuser in your workspace, create a roll-on applicator for a quick pick-me-up, or even incorporate them into a morning meditation practice to set a focused and energized tone for the day.

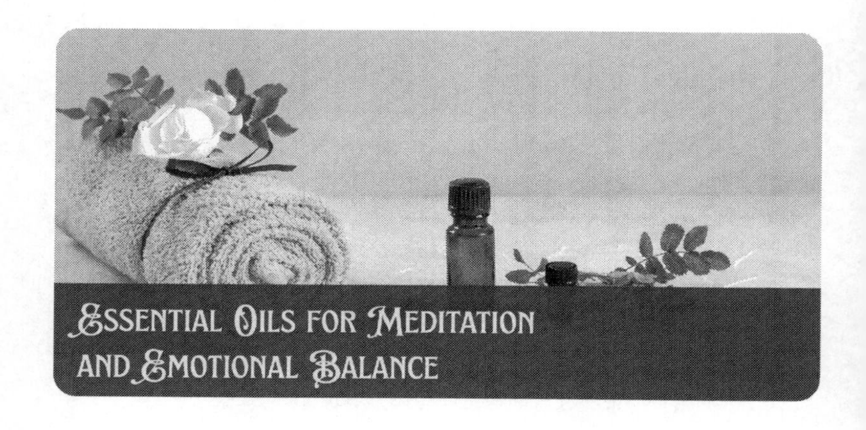

Essential Oils for Meditation and Emotional Balance

Meditation is a powerful practice for achieving emotional balance and inner peace. Essential oils can deepen the meditative experience by grounding the mind and creating a serene environment that allows for introspection and spiritual connection. When creating blends for meditation, focus on oils that promote stillness, enhance spiritual awareness, and support emotional balance.

Frankincense, often called the "oil of spirituality," has been used in religious and spiritual ceremonies for centuries. Its rich, resinous aroma can help calm the mind, deepen the breath and facilitate a meditative state. When combined with sandalwood, another spiritually grounding oil, the blend creates a sacred atmosphere perfect for meditation and emotional healing. Sandalwood's warm, woody scent is known to quiet mental chatter and promote a sense of presence and mindfulness.

For emotional balance, Geranium and Patchouli make a powerful pair. Geranium has a sweet, floral scent that is uplifting and harmonizing, helping to stabilize emotions and promote a sense of calm. It is particularly effective in reducing feelings of anxiety and promoting a sense of well-being. Patchouli, with its deep, earthy aroma, is grounding and centering, making it ideal for balancing emotions and alleviating feelings of restlessness. Together, Geranium and Patchouli can be used to create a blend that brings a sense of harmony to the mind and heart.

Lavender, while commonly associated with relaxation, is also highly effective in promoting emotional balance. When combined with vetiver and bergamot, it creates a soothing blend that helps release pent-up emotions and promotes a sense of inner peace. Vetiver's grounding properties anchor the mind, while Bergamot uplifts the spirit, creating a well-rounded blend that is both calming and rejuvenating. This combination can be diffused during meditation or used as an anointing oil on the temples and wrists to promote emotional stability.

For those seeking a more spiritual and enlightening experience, myrrh and clary sage can be used together to open the mind and facilitate deeper spiritual insights. Myrrh has a rich, balsamic scent that promotes a sense of timelessness and reverence, while Clary Sage enhances intuition and emotional release. This blend can be used in a personal meditation practice or during rituals to create a sacred space.

Whether you are seeking to calm anxiety, improve focus, or achieve emotional balance, essential oil blends can be a powerful tool in your self-care and wellness practice. By understanding the properties and effects of different oils, you can create personalized blends that support your mental and emotional well-being and bring a sense of harmony and peace to your daily life.

CHAPTER 4

Immune-Boosting and Respiratory Support Oils

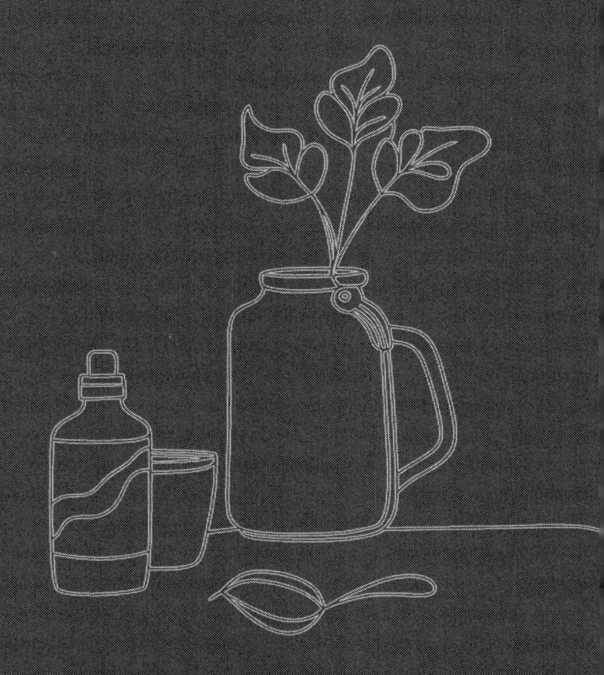

The health of our immune system is vital to our overall well-being, especially in the face of seasonal colds, flu, and other illnesses. Essential oils offer powerful properties that can help boost immunity and support respiratory function. This chapter explores several essential oils known for their immune-boosting and respiratory-supporting properties, and provides you with the knowledge to incorporate these natural remedies into your health routine.

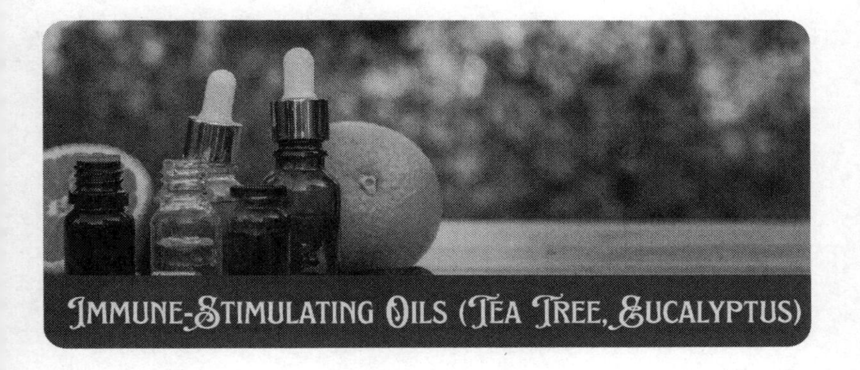

Immune-Stimulating Oils (Tea Tree, Eucalyptus)

Essential oils have been used for centuries for their medicinal properties, particularly their ability to support the immune system. Among the most revered immune-boosting oils are tea tree and eucalyptus, each of which offers unique benefits that can help strengthen the body's defenses against infection and disease.

Tea tree oil, derived from the leaves of the Melaleuca alternifolia tree native to Australia, is celebrated for its powerful antibacterial, antiviral and antifungal properties. Its unique composition contains compounds such as terpinen-4-ol, which is responsible for many of its therapeutic effects. Tea tree oil works by disrupting the cell membranes of bacteria and viruses, rendering them ineffective and helping the body fight off infections. This oil is particularly useful in preventing colds and flu because it can be applied topically to the skin or diffused into the air to purify the environment. In addition, Tea Tree Oil can be incorporated into natural cleaning products to enhance their antimicrobial properties, effectively reducing the presence of germs in the home.

Eucalyptus oil, known for its refreshing and invigorating scent, is another essential oil that significantly boosts immunity. It contains eucalyptol, a compound known for its ability to support respiratory health. Eucalyptus oil has expectorant properties, helping to clear mucus from the airways and making it easier to breathe during times of congestion. Its ability to boost the immune response makes it especially effective during cold and flu season. When diffused, eucalyptus oil can create a calming atmosphere while purifying the air. When diluted in a carrier oil, it can be applied topically to the chest and back to ease breathing and relieve sinus pressure.

Creating a blend that combines tea tree and eucalyptus oils can create a synergistic effect, enhancing the immune-boosting benefits of both oils. This powerful combination can be used in a diffuser to purify the air and support respiratory health, especially in common areas. In addition, using these oils in a warm bath or steam inhalation can provide immediate relief from respiratory discomfort, making breathing easier and promoting relaxation.

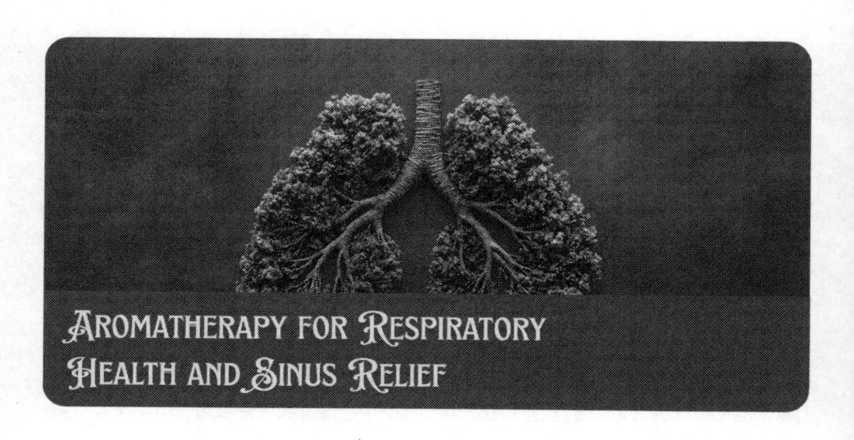

Aromatherapy is a holistic healing practice that harnesses the power of essential oils to promote health and wellness. When it comes to respiratory health, certain essential oils can provide significant relief from congestion, sinus pressure, and other respiratory issues. Incorporating these oils into your self-care routine can support overall respiratory function and comfort.

One of the most effective approaches to respiratory support is to use essential oils in a diffuser. Oils such as peppermint, thyme, and rosemary can create a soothing and invigorating atmosphere that eases breathing. Peppermint oil, with its cooling menthol properties, is particularly beneficial for clearing the nasal passages and soothing irritated airways. When diffused, peppermint oil not only promotes alertness and focus, but also helps alleviate symptoms of respiratory discomfort, making it a popular choice during the colder months.

Thyme oil is another excellent choice for respiratory health. It has powerful antimicrobial and expectorant properties, making it effective in fighting coughs and colds. Thyme oil can help reduce mucus production and assist the body in fighting infection. When combined with eucalyptus and peppermint in a diffuser, this blend can provide significant relief during times of respiratory distress.

Rosemary oil, with its woody and herbaceous aroma, also plays a role in respiratory health. It is known for its ability to improve circulation and stimulate the immune system. Inhaling rosemary oil can help reduce respiratory infections and soothe coughs. Combining rosemary oil with lavender can create a calming blend that promotes relaxation while supporting respiratory function.

In addition to diffusion, steam inhalation is an effective way to deliver the benefits of essential oils directly to the respiratory system. To perform steam inhalation, simply fill a bowl with hot water, add a few drops of your chosen essential oils, cover your head with a towel, and lean over the bowl to inhale the steam. This technique helps open the nasal passages, relieve congestion, and provide immediate relief.

Aromatherapy can also be applied topically to promote respiratory health. A simple chest rub can be made by diluting essential oils such as eucalyptus, peppermint, and tea tree oil in a carrier oil. This mixture can be massaged into the chest and back to help open the airways and ease breathing. For added benefit, a warm compress soaked in a diluted blend of essential oils can be placed on the chest for a soothing effect.

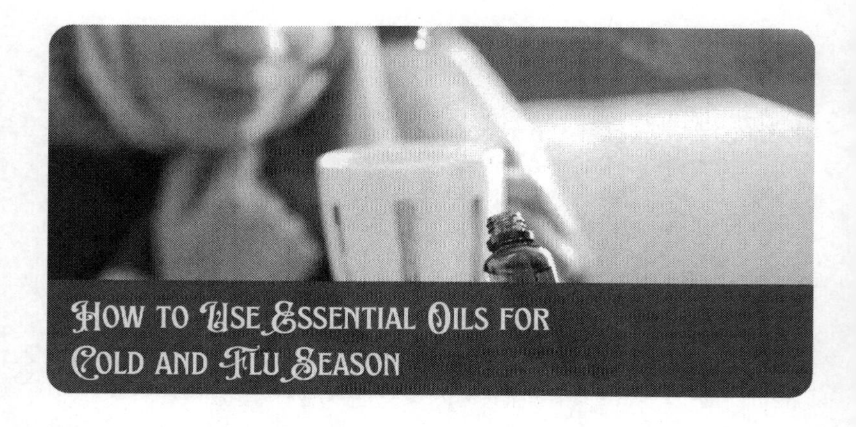

How to Use Essential Oils for Cold and Flu Season

Cold and flu season can be especially challenging, but essential oils can provide a natural and effective way to support your immune system and boost your body's defenses against these common illnesses. Understanding how to properly use essential oils during this time can empower you to take proactive measures to maintain your health.

The first step in using essential oils during cold and flu season is prevention. Regular diffusion of essential oils known for their immune-boosting properties, such as tea tree, eucalyptus, and lemon, can help purify the air and reduce the presence of airborne pathogens. This practice can be especially beneficial in common areas where viruses can easily spread. Creating a protective environment by incorporating these oils into your daily routine can help keep your family healthy.

When symptoms arise, essential oils can be used in a variety of ways to provide relief. For example, a blend of eucalyptus and peppermint can be used in vapor inhalation to clear the nasal passages and promote easier breathing. This blend can also be diluted and applied topically to the chest to help relieve congestion.

For sore throats, a soothing throat gargle can be made by mixing a few drops of lemon essential oil with warm water and salt. Gargling with this mixture can help reduce inflammation and relieve discomfort. Lemon oil also has antiviral properties that can help fight infections.

A warm bath infused with essential oils can also provide relief during cold and flu season. Adding a few drops of lavender, eucalyptus, or chamomile oil to a warm bath can promote relaxation and help relieve muscle tension associated with illness. The steam from the bath can also help clear the nasal passages for added comfort.

Finally, incorporating essential oils into your wellness routine can enhance overall immune support. Drinking herbal teas infused with immune-boosting oils can help strengthen your body. For example, adding a drop of thyme essential oil to warm honey and lemon tea can create a soothing beverage that supports respiratory health and provides relief from cold symptoms.

By understanding the different uses of essential oils, you can create a comprehensive plan for staying healthy during cold and flu season. These natural remedies not only support the immune system, but also provide a sense of comfort and well-being, making them valuable additions to your self-care regimen.

CHAPTER 5

Beauty and Skin Care with Essential Oils

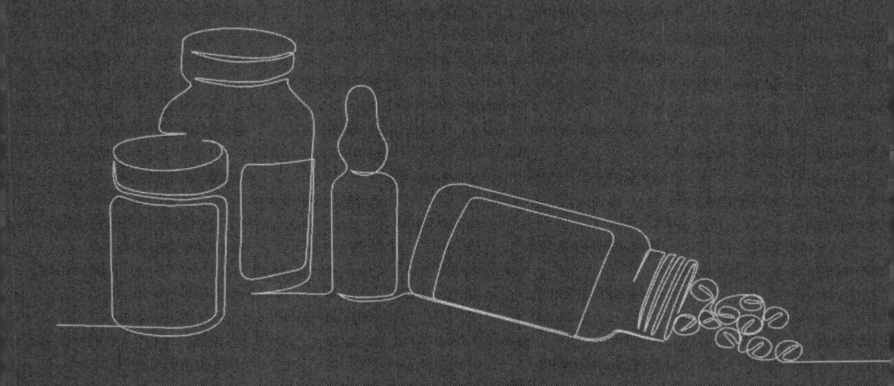

Essential oils have transcended their traditional uses and found a prominent place in the beauty and skin care industry. Their powerful properties can improve skin health, rejuvenate hair, and provide a natural alternative to synthetic products. In this chapter, we will explore how to incorporate essential oils into your daily beauty routine, focusing on their benefits for glowing skin and healthy hair, creating nourishing facial oils and cleansing balms, and effectively treating issues such as acne, scars, and blemishes.

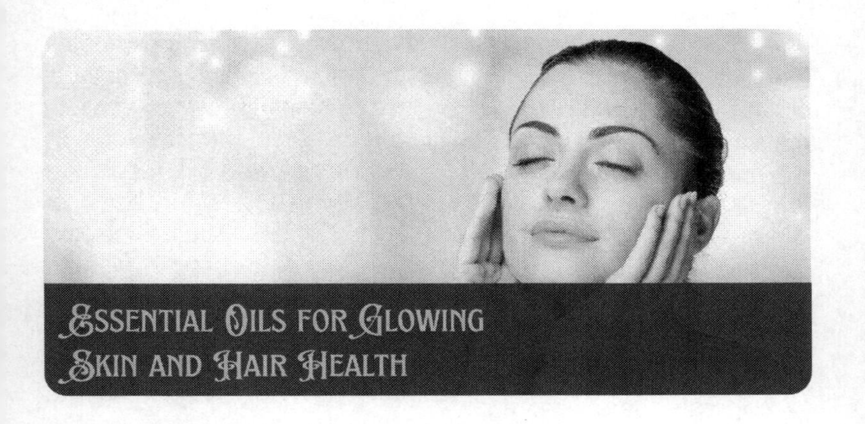

Essential Oils for Glowing Skin and Hair Health

The quest for glowing skin and vibrant hair has led many to turn to nature for solutions. Essential oils, with their concentrated botanical properties, offer remarkable benefits for both skin and hair, promoting youthful appearance and overall health.

One of the standout essential oils for skin health is frankincense. Known for its anti-aging properties, frankincense helps reduce the appearance of fine lines and wrinkles while promoting even skin tone. It is rich in boswellic acids, which have anti-inflammatory properties, making it effective for soothing irritated skin. Frankincense can be combined with a carrier oil, such as jojoba or sweet almond oil, and applied to the skin to improve elasticity and promote a youthful glow. Regular use can result in a noticeable improvement in skin texture, resulting in a healthy and radiant appearance.

Lavender oil is another excellent choice for skin care. Its calming and soothing properties make it suitable for all skin types, including sensitive and acne-prone skin. Lavender is known for its ability to promote healing, reduce redness and prevent breakouts. Incorporating lavender oil into a nighttime skincare routine can help calm inflamed skin and promote a balanced complexion. In addition, its pleasant scent can promote relaxation, making it a perfect addition to a self-care ritual.

For hair health, rosemary essential oil is a powerful ally. It stimulates hair follicles, promoting hair growth and reducing hair loss. Rosemary oil also increases blood flow to the scalp, helping to nourish the hair roots. By adding a few drops of rosemary oil to your regular shampoo or creating a hair mask with a carrier oil, you can support healthier hair growth and add shine. The refreshing scent of rosemary also helps to invigorate the senses during your hair care routine.

Tea Tree Oil is known for its antiseptic properties and can effectively treat scalp problems such as dandruff and itchiness. Its antifungal properties combat the yeast that often contributes to dandruff, while its soothing nature helps to relieve irritation. When diluted with a carrier oil and massaged into the scalp, tea tree oil can help restore balance, leaving the scalp healthy and the hair looking vibrant.

Combining essential oils such as frankincense, lavender, rosemary, and tea tree can create a powerful beauty regimen that promotes healthy skin and hair. Incorporating these oils into your daily routine not only enhances your appearance, but also provides a holistic approach to self-care, allowing you to reap the benefits of nature's bounty.

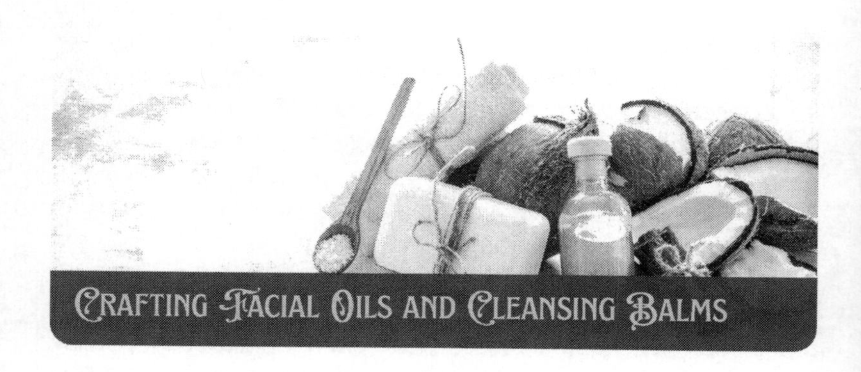

Crafting Facial Oils and Cleansing Balms

Creating your own facial oils and cleansing balms is a rewarding way to tailor skincare products to your unique needs while harnessing the power of essential oils. These homemade preparations allow you to control the ingredients, ensuring that they are free of harmful additives and suitable for your skin type.

Facial oils are a fantastic way to nourish and hydrate the skin. When creating a facial oil blend, it's important to choose a carrier oil that matches your skin type. For example, jojoba oil is great for oily and combination skin because it mimics the skin's natural sebum and helps regulate oil production. For dry skin, sweet almond or argan oil can provide the necessary hydration without clogging pores.

Once you've chosen your carrier oil, you can enhance its benefits by adding essential oils that promote skin health. For a rejuvenating blend, consider adding a few drops of rose essential oil, known for its moisturizing and anti-inflammatory properties. In addition to moisturizing, rose oil helps reduce redness and promotes even skin tone. A few drops of geranium oil can further balance oil production while providing a beautiful floral scent.

To use the facial oil, simply massage a few drops onto cleansed skin each evening before bed. This not only moisturizes, but also provides an opportunity for self-care and relaxation, allowing the oils to absorb overnight and reveal a refreshed complexion in the morning.

In addition to facial oils, making your own cleansing balms is an effective way to remove makeup and cleanse the skin without stripping it of its natural oils. A simple cleansing balm can be made with coconut oil as the base, combined with beeswax for texture and essential oils for added benefits. For example, adding lavender oil can enhance the calming effect, while chamomile oil can soothe irritated skin.

To make the balm, melt the coconut oil and beeswax together, then remove from the heat and allow to cool slightly before adding the essential oils. Once mixed, pour the balm into small jars and allow to solidify. This balm can be used by warming a small amount between the palms of your hands and gently massaging it onto the skin to effectively dissolve makeup and impurities. The balm is then wiped away with a warm cloth, leaving the skin clean and nourished.

The process of creating facial oils and cleansing balms is not only empowering, but also allows for a personalized skin care routine that aligns with your values. By using high-quality ingredients and essential oils, you can create effective products that enhance your natural beauty while promoting skin health.

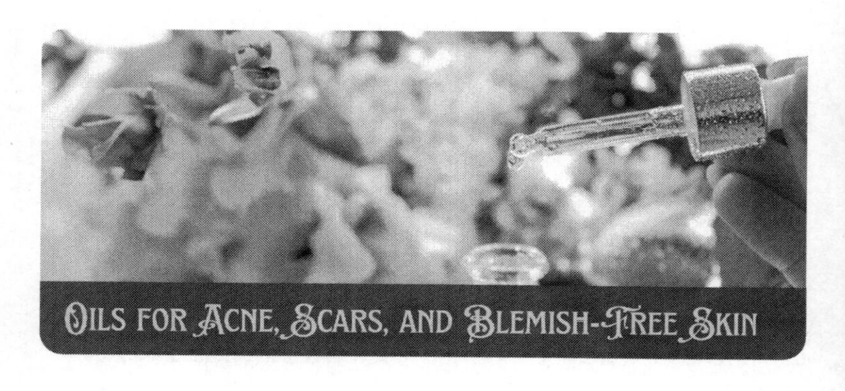

Oils for Acne, Scars, and Blemish-Free Skin

Managing acne and scarring can be a frustrating journey, but essential oils offer a natural alternative to conventional treatments. With their antibacterial, anti-inflammatory, and healing properties, certain essential oils can effectively treat breakouts and promote clearer, healthier skin.

Tea tree oil, known for its powerful antibacterial properties, is a staple in acne treatments. It targets the bacteria that contribute to breakouts while reducing inflammation and redness. Applying diluted tea tree oil directly to blemishes can help dry them out and speed the healing process. When combined with lavender oil, known for its calming properties, the blend can soothe the skin and prevent further irritation, making it ideal for those with sensitive skin.

Another excellent choice for acne-prone skin is lavender essential oil. Its ability to reduce redness and promote healing makes it a valuable addition to any acne treatment routine. Lavender oil can also help balance oil production and reduce stress, which can often exacerbate breakouts. Incorporating lavender into a facial oil or applying it to affected areas can help reduce the severity of acne.

In addition to treating active breakouts, essential oils can be beneficial in minimizing the appearance of scars. Boswellia oil is particularly known for its skin-regenerating properties. It promotes the regeneration of healthy skin cells, helping to fade scars and improve skin texture over time. A combination of frankincense and helichrysum oil - a powerful oil known for its wound-healing and skin-rejuvenating properties - can create a powerful scar treatment blend. This blend can be diluted in a carrier oil and applied daily to scarred areas for best results.

For those struggling with hyperpigmentation or blemishes, carrot seed oil can be a beneficial addition to your skin care regimen. Rich in antioxidants and vitamins A and E, carrot seed oil promotes cell turnover and helps improve skin tone. This oil can be blended with a light carrier oil and used as a spot treatment, or incorporated into a daily facial oil to gradually reduce the appearance of dark spots.

The versatility of essential oils in addressing skin concerns means that they can be incorporated into a holistic skin care routine. By selecting oils that specifically address your unique skin concerns and using them regularly, you can create a natural, effective approach to achieving clear, radiant skin.

In conclusion, essential oils play a multifaceted role in beauty and skin care, providing effective, natural solutions to a variety of concerns. Whether you create your own oils, balms, or ointments, the potential for healing and rejuvenation is vast. By harnessing the power of nature, you can take a holistic approach to self-care that supports both your physical and emotional well-being.

CHAPTER 6

Natural Household Cleaning with Essential Oils

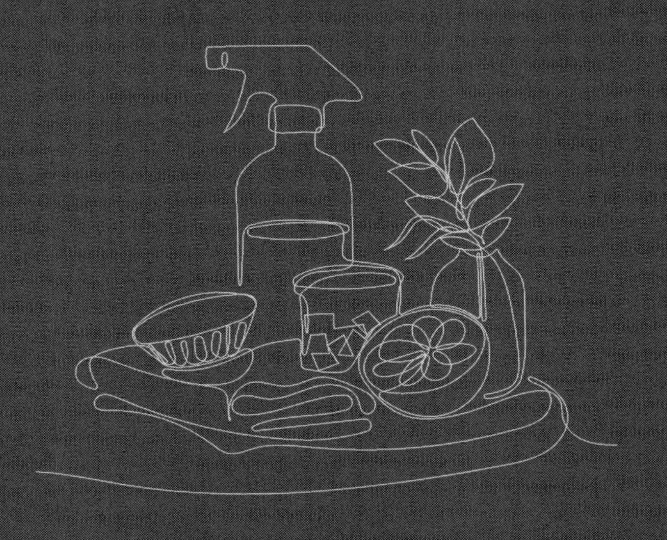

At a time when many are becoming increasingly aware of the potential dangers associated with conventional cleaning products, the shift to natural alternatives has gained momentum. Essential oils offer a powerful and versatile solution for maintaining a clean and healthy home without the harsh chemicals that can pose risks to our health and the environment.

This chapter explores how essential oils can be incorporated into household cleaning routines, with a focus on creating non-toxic cleaning solutions, ensuring a fresh environment, and creating multi-purpose blends to meet various cleaning needs.

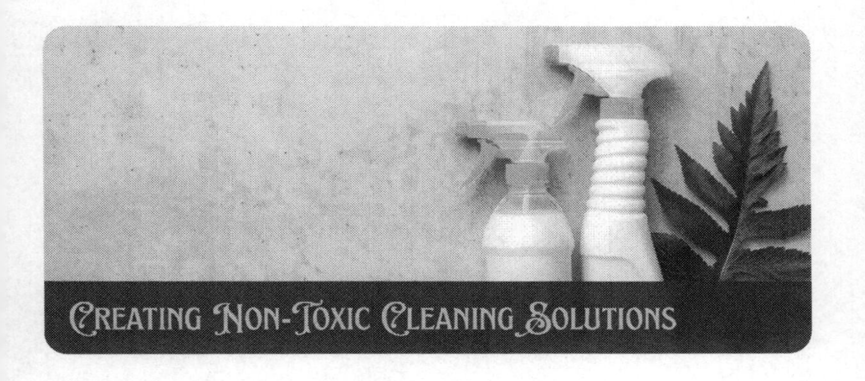

Creating Non-Toxic Cleaning Solutions

Making your own non-toxic cleaning solutions with essential oils is not only an effective way to keep your home clean, but also a step toward a healthier living environment.

Many commercial cleaning products are loaded with synthetic fragrances, preservatives, and toxic chemicals that can irritate the skin, respiratory system, and even contribute to long-term health problems. By making your own cleaning solutions, you can ensure that your home is free of these harmful substances, while also benefiting from the natural antimicrobial and antiseptic properties of essential oils.

The base of most homemade cleaning solutions can be a simple combination of distilled water, white vinegar, and essential oils. White vinegar is a natural disinfectant that effectively cuts through dirt and eliminates odors. It can be combined with essential oils to enhance its cleaning power and add pleasant fragrances to your home.

For example, a basic all-purpose cleaner can be made by mixing one cup of water, one cup of white vinegar, and about 20-30 drops of essential oils such as tea tree, lemon, or lavender. Tea tree oil is particularly effective due to its strong antibacterial and antifungal properties, making it ideal for disinfecting surfaces. Lemon oil, on the other hand, not only adds a refreshing scent, but also has natural grease cutting properties, making it perfect for kitchens and dining areas.

For a more specialized cleaner, consider making a glass cleaner with distilled water, vinegar, and a few drops of peppermint or eucalyptus oil. This mixture not only cleans and polishes glass surfaces, but also leaves a fresh, invigorating scent. In addition, the use of essential oils such as orange or grapefruit can enhance the cleaning experience while providing powerful antimicrobial benefits.

As you create your non-toxic cleaning solutions, it's important to remember proper storage and labeling. Store your homemade cleaners in dark glass bottles to protect the integrity of the essential oils, as sunlight can degrade their potency. Clearly label each bottle to avoid confusion and ensure safe use, especially if there are children or pets in the household.

Switching to natural cleaning solutions empowers you to take control of your environment and ensure that your home is not only clean, but also a safe space for your family. By choosing essential oils as your cleaning allies, you are promoting a healthier, more sustainable lifestyle.

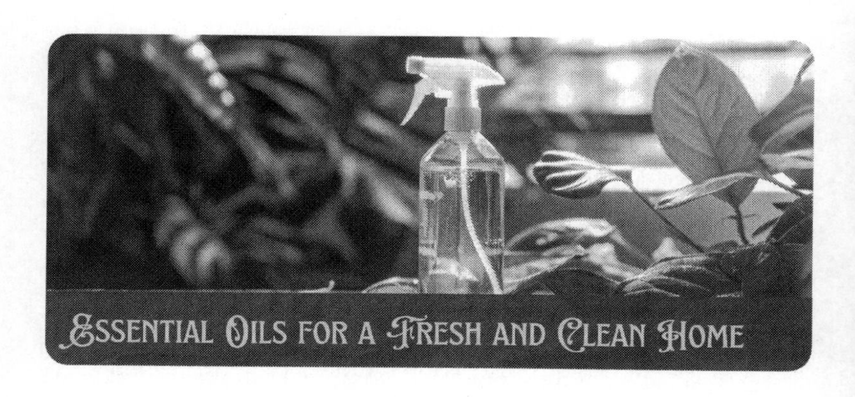

Essential Oils for a Fresh and Clean Home

Creating a fresh and inviting atmosphere in the home goes beyond simply cleaning surfaces to maintaining an environment that promotes well-being and positivity. Essential oils are excellent allies in achieving this goal, offering natural fragrances that lift the spirit while providing additional cleaning benefits.

One of the most popular essential oils for freshening up a home is lemon oil. Its bright, citrusy scent is instantly uplifting and has powerful antibacterial properties, making it perfect for combating unpleasant odors.

Lemon oil can be used in a variety of ways, from adding a few drops to your cleaning solutions to incorporating it into a diffuser. When diffused, lemon oil not only freshens the air, but can also improve mood and concentration, creating a pleasant atmosphere for work or relaxation.

Another excellent option is lavender oil, which is known for its calming and soothing properties. Lavender not only freshens the air but also promotes relaxation, making it ideal for bedrooms and living spaces.

A simple yet effective way to use lavender is to add a few drops to a cotton ball and place it in closets or drawers to infuse fabrics with its delightful scent. Alternatively, you can make a lavender laundry spray by mixing water with a few drops of lavender oil in a spray bottle. This can be used on bedding, upholstery, and even in the air to create a calm and inviting atmosphere.

Peppermint oil adds a refreshing and invigorating scent that can help clear the air and energize a room. Its strong aroma is effective at masking unpleasant odors, making it an excellent choice for kitchens and bathrooms. A few drops of peppermint oil can be added to your mop water or cleaning solutions for added freshness. When diffused, peppermint oil can help stimulate the mind and improve concentration, creating a motivating environment for productivity.

For a natural air freshener, consider combining several essential oils known for their cleansing properties. A blend of tea tree, eucalyptus, and rosemary can be combined with water in a spray bottle to create a refreshing room spray that purifies the air and lifts the mood. This blend not only fights odors, but also contributes to a cleaner atmosphere by helping to neutralize airborne pathogens.

Using essential oils for a fresher home goes beyond adding pleasant scents. Their natural antibacterial and antiviral properties can help improve indoor air quality and create a healthier living environment. By incorporating these oils into your cleaning and freshening routines, you will cultivate a space that nurtures both body and mind.

Multi-Purpose Cleaning Blends and Air Fresheners

Creating multi-purpose cleaning blends with essential oils allows you to streamline your cleaning routine while maximizing effectiveness and minimizing clutter. These versatile blends can tackle a variety of surfaces and tasks, from disinfecting counters to freshening laundry, making them invaluable in any household.

A well-rounded multi-purpose cleaner can be created using a combination of essential oils that offer both cleaning and aromatic benefits. A blend of lemon, tea tree and lavender creates a powerful yet pleasant cleaning solution.

The natural acidity of lemon helps cut through grease and grime, while tea tree oil offers its powerful antimicrobial properties. Lavender, with its soothing scent, not only soothes the mind but also leaves surfaces smelling fresh and inviting. To make this blend, mix one cup of distilled water, one cup of vinegar, and about 10 drops of each essential oil in a spray bottle. This cleaner can be used on countertops, kitchen surfaces, and even in the bathroom for a clean and fragrant environment.

For those looking for an all-natural way to freshen laundry, consider adding essential oils directly to your wash cycle. Adding a few drops of your favorite essential oils, such as eucalyptus or lavender, to your laundry detergent can give your clothes a delightful scent.

Eucalyptus oil also has antimicrobial properties that help keep laundry fresh, making it a convenient choice for towels and bedding. Alternatively, you can make reusable dryer balls by adding a few drops of essential oil to wool dryer balls before throwing them in with your laundry. Not only will this reduce drying time, but it will also add a natural scent to your clothes.

To maintain a fresh-smelling home without relying on synthetic air fresheners, consider making your own essential oil air freshener. Combining water and essential oils in a spray bottle allows for easy spritzing throughout the home.

The combination of grapefruit and rosemary provides a refreshing and invigorating scent that can lift your spirits. This blend can be sprinkled in common areas such as living rooms or entryways to create a welcoming atmosphere.

Another way to enhance your environment with essential oils is to use a potpourri blend. Create a mixture of dried herbs, flowers, and essential oils to make a natural air freshener.

Dried lavender, rose petals, and a few drops of bergamot oil create a beautifully scented potpourri that can be placed in decorative bowls around the home. This not only adds visual appeal, but also fills the air with soothing scents.

By using multi-purpose cleaning blends and air fresheners made with essential oils, you can simplify your cleaning routine while promoting a healthy, welcoming home environment.

The versatility of essential oils offers endless possibilities, allowing you to customize your cleaning products to suit your family's needs and preferences. Embracing these natural solutions not only enhances your home, but also supports a lifestyle based on wellness and sustainability.

CHAPTER 7

Everyday Rituals with Essential Oils

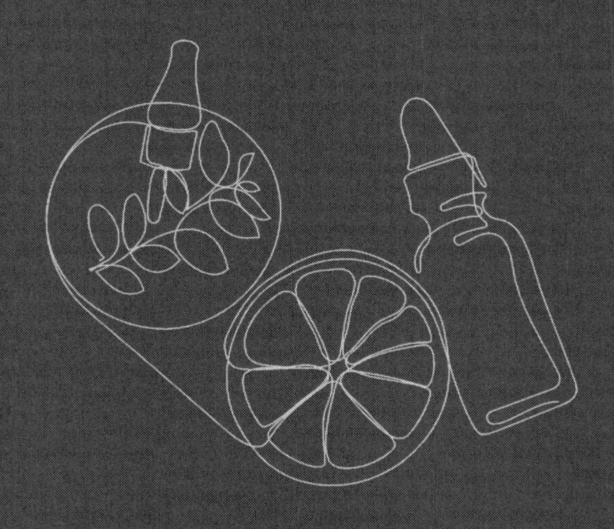

Incorporating essential oils into your daily rituals can transform ordinary routines into extraordinary self-care practices. These powerful plant extracts not only provide therapeutic benefits, but also enhance your overall well-being by creating an atmosphere of calm, rejuvenation, and mindfulness. This chapter explores how to weave aromatherapy into the fabric of daily life, emphasizing its applications in self-care routines, massage, bathing, and creating a personal spa experience at home.

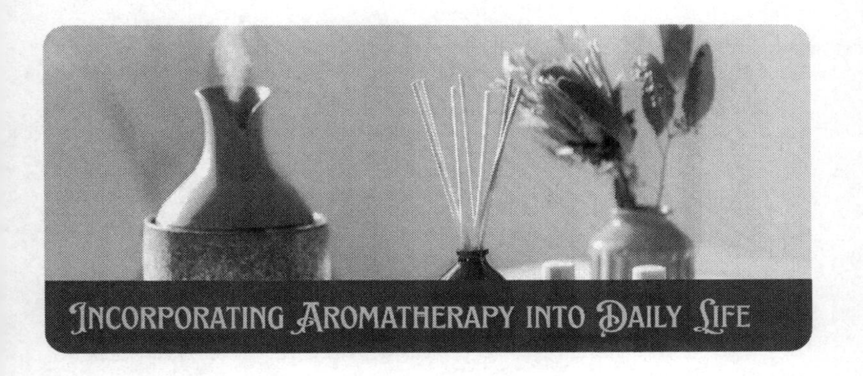

Incorporating Aromatherapy into Daily Life

Aromatherapy is a powerful tool that can enrich our daily lives by promoting relaxation, focus, and emotional balance. By consciously incorporating essential oils into various aspects of your routine, you can create an environment that supports your mental and physical health.

One of the easiest ways to start is with a diffuser. By placing a diffuser in your living space, you can fill the air with the uplifting scents of essential oils throughout the day. For morning motivation, consider diffusing a blend of citrus oils such as lemon, orange, and grapefruit.

The bright, invigorating scents of these oils can help awaken your senses, improve your mood, and promote alertness as you start your day. As you prepare breakfast or get ready for work, the aroma can serve as a refreshing reminder to set positive intentions.

Throughout the day, essential oils can also be used as personal inhalers. A small inhaler can be filled with a blend of your favorite oils to provide an instant aromatic boost whenever you need it. For example, a combination of peppermint and rosemary is great for increasing focus and reducing fatigue during busy work hours. Simply take a few deep breaths from the inhaler to invigorate your mind and sharpen your focus.

Even in your workspace, essential oils can increase productivity and reduce stress. A drop of lavender or chamomile on a cotton ball in your desk drawer can create a calming atmosphere, helping to ease anxiety during hectic workdays. In addition, creating an essential oil roller with calming oils such as frankincense or bergamot can be applied to pulse points for an on-the-go relaxation tool.

In the evening, aromatherapy can help you transition to a more serene atmosphere. Consider diffusing calming oils such as cedarwood, ylang-ylang, or vetiver to signal your body that it's time to relax.

You can also create a calming bedtime routine by incorporating essential oils into your skincare routine. Adding a few drops of lavender or chamomile oil to your nighttime moisturizer can help you relax and prepare for a restful night's sleep.

By intentionally incorporating aromatherapy into your daily life, you can foster a greater sense of well-being, create balance, and cultivate a nurturing environment that supports your mental and emotional health.

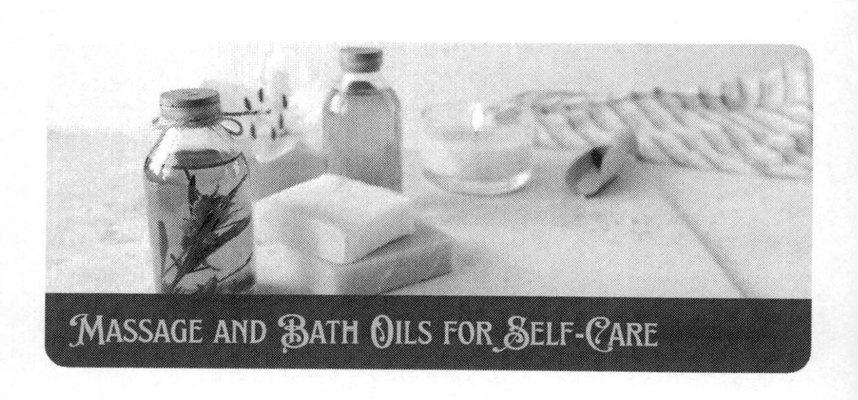

Massage and Bath Oils for Self-Care

Massage and bathing are timeless practices that promote relaxation and rejuvenation. Infusing these self-care rituals with essential oils not only enhances their benefits, but also creates a sensory experience that nurtures both the body and mind. Creating your own massage oils and bath blends allows you to personalize your self-care routine while tapping into the therapeutic properties of essential oils.

To create a soothing massage oil, start with a carrier oil that suits your skin type, such as sweet almond, jojoba, or fractionated coconut oil. These oils provide a smooth glide while nourishing the skin.

The general rule for dilution is to use about 3-5% essential oil in your carrier oil. For a calming massage blend, consider combining lavender and chamomile essential oils. Both oils are known for their relaxing properties, making them ideal for unwinding after a long day.

Mixing approximately 10-15 drops of lavender and chamomile oil into one ounce of carrier oil creates a calming blend that can help soothe sore muscles and promote relaxation. This oil can be used for self-massage or as part of a shared experience with a partner to enhance emotional connection and intimacy.

For those seeking invigorating energy, consider creating a blend with peppermint and rosemary essential oils. This combination can stimulate circulation and invigorate the senses, making it perfect for a morning massage or post-exercise recovery. Dilute the oils in a carrier oil and use during a muscle-relaxing massage to promote vitality and reduce fatigue.

Bathing is another extraordinary way to incorporate essential oils into your self-care routine. A warm bath infused with essential oils can transform a simple soak into a luxurious, therapeutic experience.

When preparing a bath, start with a base of Epsom or sea salts, which can help detoxify the body and relieve muscle tension. Add about 10-15 drops of essential oils, such as lavender for relaxation or eucalyptus for respiratory support.

Creating a calming bath oil can also be beneficial. Mix your favorite essential oils with a carrier oil and add to your bath water. Essential oils such as ylang-ylang and sandalwood not only provide a soothing scent, but also promote emotional well-being. As you soak in warm water, the steam helps release the oils into the air, enhancing your overall bathing experience.

By incorporating massage and essential oil bathing into your self-care routine, you can create a sanctuary that nurtures your body and soul. These rituals offer an opportunity to slow down, reconnect, and prioritize your well-being in a world that often demands constant movement and attention.

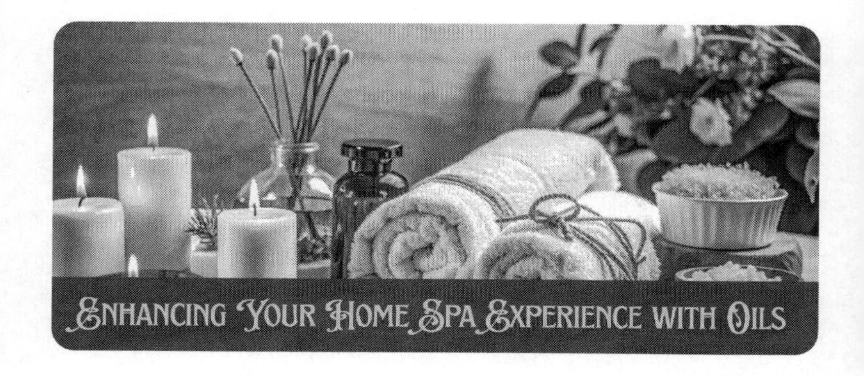

Transforming your home into a spa-like retreat is a rewarding way to prioritize self-care and relaxation. Essential oils play an important role in creating a calming and rejuvenating atmosphere, allowing you to unwind and indulge in luxurious experiences without leaving your home.

Start by creating a serene environment that invites relaxation. Dim the lights, play soft music, and remove any distractions from your room. Incorporate essential oils through diffusers, candles, or massage oils. Consider using calming oils such as lavender, bergamot, or sandalwood to set the mood. Diffusing these oils fills the room with a delightful aroma, creating a peaceful atmosphere conducive to relaxation and introspection.

Creating a spa experience often includes facial treatments. You can create a soothing facial steam by boiling water and adding a few drops of essential oils such as eucalyptus or chamomile.

The steam opens the pores, allowing the oils to penetrate the skin more effectively. Drape a towel over your head while leaning over the bowl to create a tent and inhale deeply as the steam envelops your face. This treatment not only refreshes the skin, but also helps clear the sinuses and promotes relaxation.

Another great way to enhance your home spa experience is with a foot soak. Fill a sink with warm water and add Epsom salts along with a few drops of essential oils such as peppermint or tea tree. The Epsom salts help draw out toxins, while the essential oils provide a soothing effect. After soaking your feet, you can follow up with a gentle foot massage using a nourishing oil infused with soothing essential oils.

To elevate your self-care ritual, consider creating a DIY facial mask using natural ingredients and essential oils. For a revitalizing mask, mix honey, yogurt, and a few drops of lavender oil. The honey acts as a natural moisturizer, while the yogurt provides gentle exfoliation and hydration. Apply this mask while enjoying a relaxing moment in your freshly scented room and allow it to work its magic for 15-20 minutes before rinsing off.

Incorporating essential oils into your home spa routine not only enhances the sensory experience, but also promotes emotional and physical well-being. Whether it's through calming massages, soothing baths, or fragrant facial treatments, these rituals offer a powerful reminder to prioritize self-care and foster a sense of peace in your daily life. Creating a nurturing environment allows you to recharge, relax, and cultivate a deeper connection with yourself, making every day a little more special.

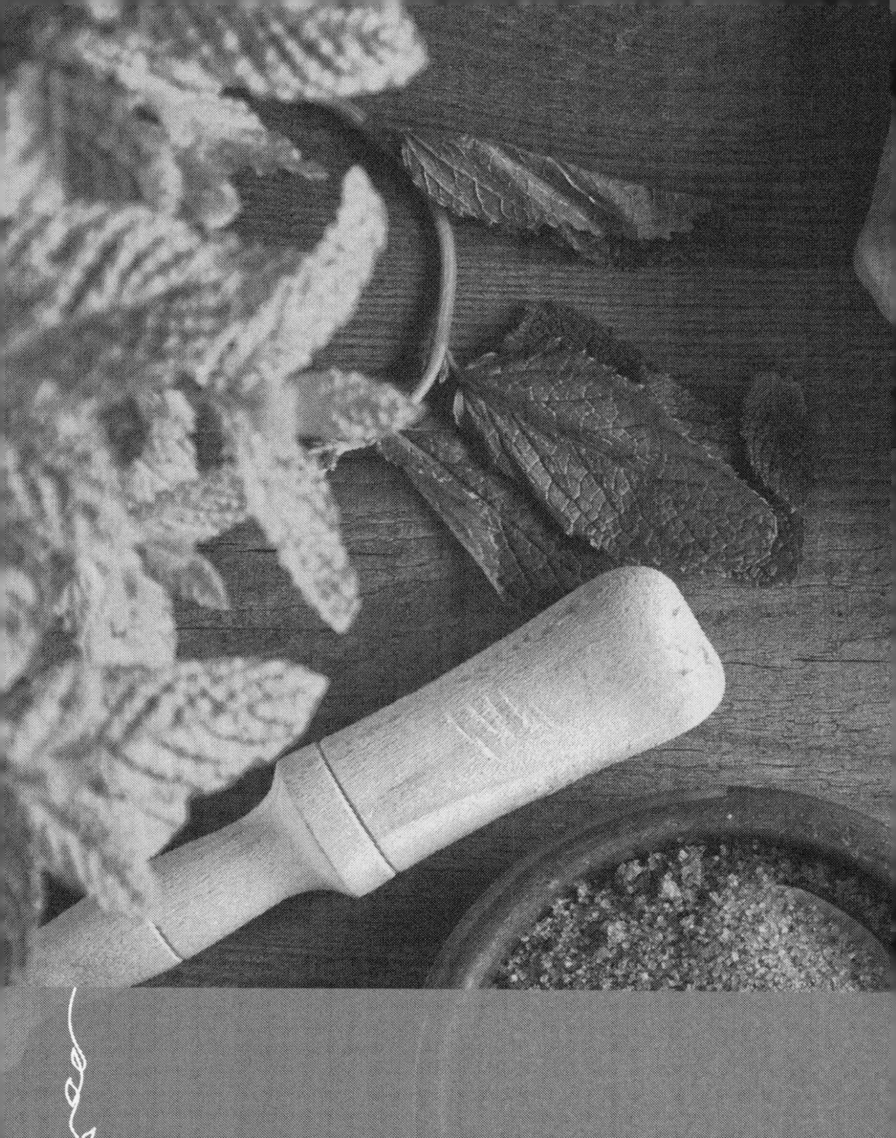

BOOK 04

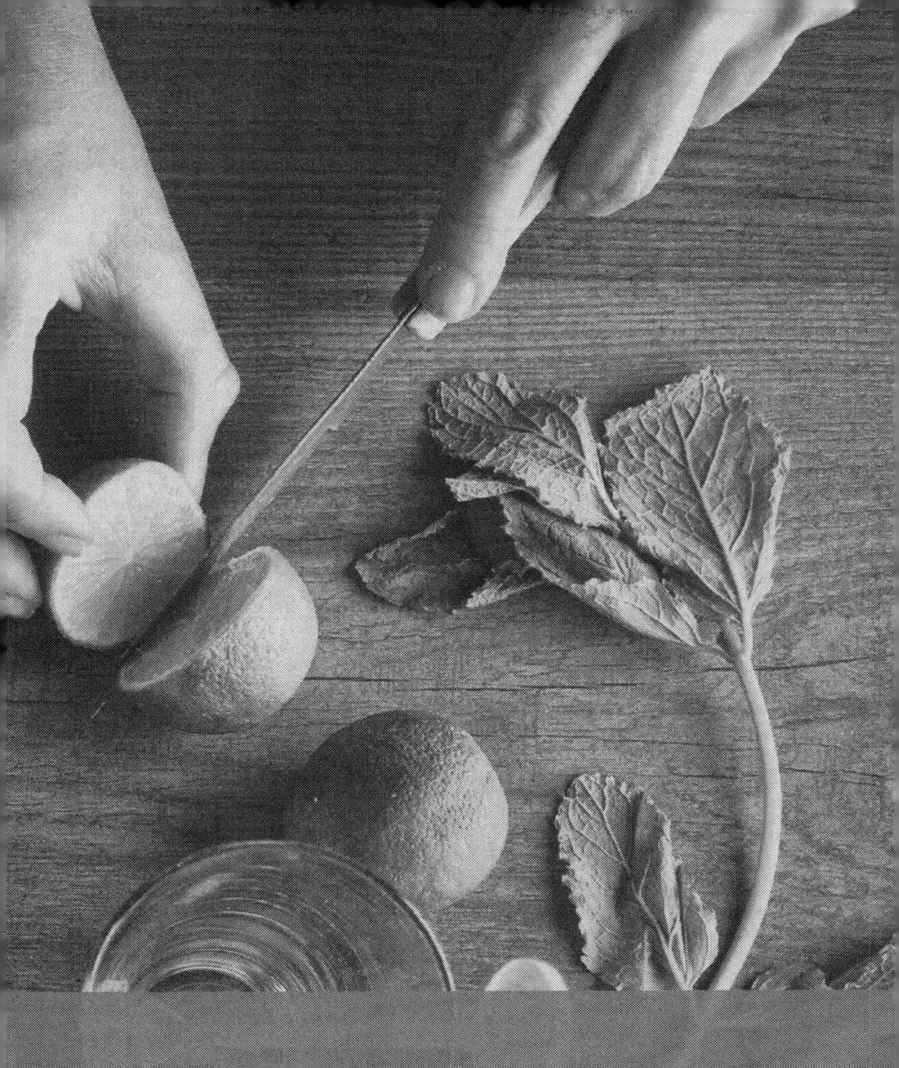

Daily Routines and Preventive Health with Herbs

Establishing a daily routine that includes herbal remedies can significantly improve overall health and well-being. By making herbs a regular part of our lives, we can help our bodies maintain balance, prevent disease, and promote vitality. This book explores how to create a daily herbal routine that fits seamlessly into your life, ensuring that you reap the many benefits herbs have to offer.

CHAPTER 1

Creating a Daily Herbal Routine

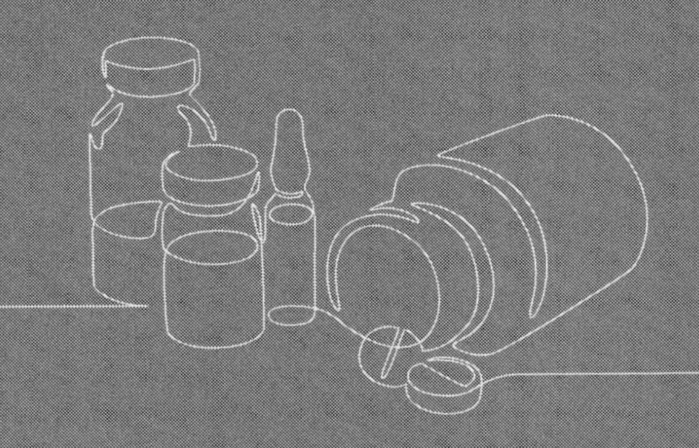

Creating a daily herbal routine is about integrating natural remedies into your life in a way that feels sustainable and supportive. By incorporating herbs into your morning, afternoon, and evening rituals, you can cultivate a lifestyle that emphasizes health and wellness. This chapter outlines the principles for creating an herbal routine that meets your needs and preferences, allowing you to take full advantage of the healing properties of herbs throughout the day.

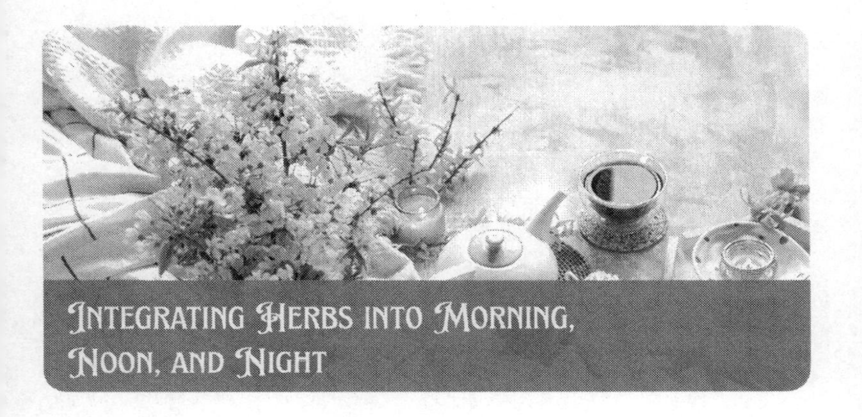

Integrating Herbs into Morning, Noon, and Night

The morning is an opportune time to set the tone for the day ahead. Beginning your day with herbal support can energize your body and mind, preparing you for the challenges ahead. One of the easiest ways to incorporate herbs into your morning routine is to enjoy an herbal tea.

For a refreshing start, consider brewing a cup of green tea with fresh ginger and lemon. Green tea is rich in antioxidants, while ginger can stimulate the digestive system and provide a gentle energy boost. Adding lemon not only enhances the flavor, but also adds vitamin C, which further supports your immune system.

As you move into the afternoon, maintaining your energy and focus becomes essential. It is important to tailor your herbal intake to your body's needs during this time. For example, if you are feeling fatigued or unfocused, incorporating an herbal tonic or adaptogenic blend can help.

Ashwagandha and Rhodiola are excellent choices for building resilience to stress and fatigue. You can prepare an herbal infusion with these adaptogens, either as a tea or in capsule form, to ensure that you have a consistent source of support throughout the day.

Evening is the perfect time to wind down and promote relaxation. Herbal remedies can help calm the mind and prepare the body for a restful night's sleep. Consider a relaxing tea blend with chamomile and valerian root, both known for their calming properties.

Chamomile is known for its mild sedative effects, making it a popular choice for promoting sleep, while valerian root has been used for centuries to relieve insomnia and anxiety. A warm cup of this herbal infusion can help signal your body that it's time to relax, making it easier to transition from the hustle and bustle of the day to a peaceful night's rest.

Incorporating herbs throughout the day can be done seamlessly by establishing simple rituals that honor your body's needs. This practice encourages mindfulness and allows you to tune into how different herbs make you feel, fostering a deeper connection with nature and your own health.

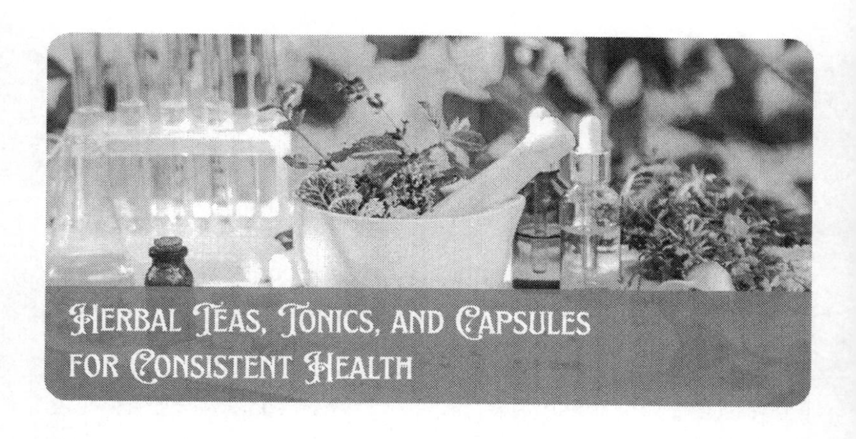

Herbal Teas, Tonics, and Capsules for Consistent Health

Consistency is key to reaping the benefits of herbal remedies. Whether consumed as teas, tonics, or capsules, these forms allow you to conveniently and effectively incorporate herbs into your daily routine. Each method offers unique benefits, so you can tailor your approach to fit your lifestyle.

Herbal teas are one of the easiest and most enjoyable ways to incorporate herbs into your daily health regimen. Brewing a pot of herbal tea can provide a moment of calm in your day, allowing you to pause and nourish your body.

For daily health maintenance, consider a blend that combines immunity-boosting herbs such as echinacea, ginger, and elderberry. These ingredients can help strengthen your body against seasonal illnesses. Drinking this tea regularly can not only support your immune system, but also encourage a ritual of self-care.

In addition to teas, herbal tonics are a concentrated way to harness the power of herbs. These tonics can be made as syrups or liquid extracts for easy consumption. For example, a daily tonic of turmeric, honey, and apple cider vinegar can help support digestion and reduce inflammation. The anti-inflammatory properties of turmeric are well documented, making this tonic an excellent addition to your health routine. Mixing these ingredients in a small glass of water each morning can serve as a powerful start to your day.

Herbal capsules are a convenient alternative for those with busy lifestyles or those who do not like the taste of certain herbs. Capsules can be filled with powdered herbs, allowing for consistent dosing without the need to brew teas or prepare tonics.

For consistent health, consider taking a daily capsule of ashwagandha or spirulina, both known for their many health benefits. Ashwagandha supports stress management and overall vitality, while spirulina is packed with nutrients and antioxidants that promote energy and well-being.

Incorporating a variety of herbal supplements into your daily health regimen ensures that you receive a wide range of benefits. Alternating teas, tonics, and capsules can keep your routine interesting and effective, ultimately promoting a lifestyle focused on health and vitality.

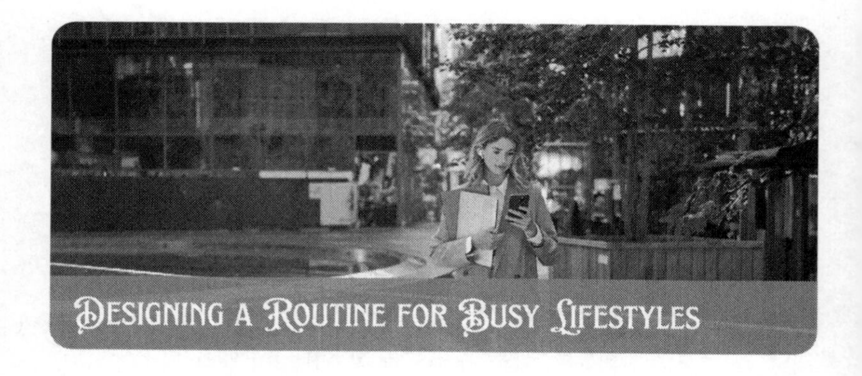

Designing a Routine for Busy Lifestyles

In our fast-paced world, finding the time to make health a priority can often feel like a challenge. However, creating a practical herbal routine that fits into a busy lifestyle is entirely achievable with a little planning and creativity. The key is to integrate herbal practices seamlessly into your existing habits so that you can maintain your well-being without overwhelming your schedule.

Start by identifying the natural rhythms of your day. Consider when you typically have time to focus on self-care-whether it's in the morning before work, during your lunch break, or in the evening when you're relaxing. Once you have a clear understanding of your daily schedule, you can tailor your herbal routine to fit these windows of time.

For example, if mornings are hectic, opt for herbal teas that can be prepared quickly. Loose leaf teas can be brewed while you shower or get dressed, so you can sip a nourishing drink as you go through your morning routine.

Consider making a large batch of herbal infusions the night before to save time in the morning. This strategy ensures that you have ready access to your favorite herbal blends without added stress.

During the day, finding moments for self-care can be as simple as incorporating herbs into your meals or snacks. For example, add fresh herbs like basil, cilantro, or parsley to your lunch salads or smoothies for an extra health boost. Plus, having herbal capsules on hand can be convenient when you need a quick energy boost or digestive support, making them an excellent choice for busy professionals.

In the evening, dedicate a few minutes to your herbal routine as a way to unwind and transition into relaxation. You can create a calming ritual by preparing a calming tea, such as chamomile or lemon balm, while engaging in a brief mindfulness practice. This combination of herbs and mindfulness can help signal to your body that it's time to relax, promoting a sense of calm as you prepare for a restful night.

Ultimately, the goal of designing an herbal routine for a busy lifestyle is to create a system that supports your health without feeling like an extra burden. By seamlessly integrating herbs into your daily activities, you can foster a proactive approach to health that enhances your well-being in the midst of life's demands. With thoughtful planning and a commitment to self-care, you can cultivate a daily routine that nourishes your body, mind, and spirit.

CHAPTER 2

Preventive Health Practices for Long-Term Wellness

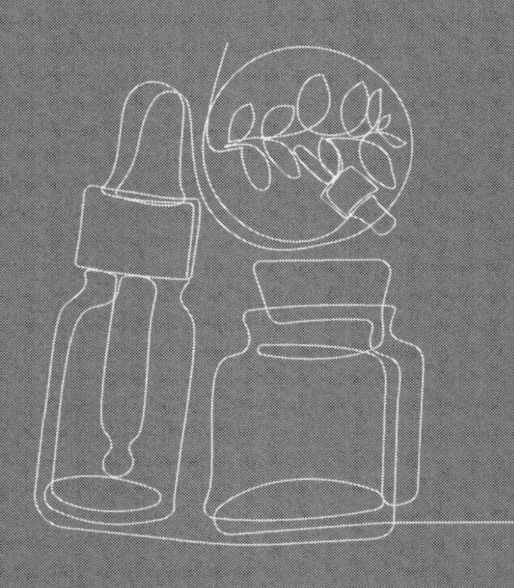

Preventive health practices are essential to maintaining overall wellness and reducing the risk of disease. A holistic approach that includes herbal remedies, teas, and tonics can support your body's natural defenses and promote a resilient immune system. This chapter explores how to build an effective herbal first aid and emergency kit, the importance of long-term immune support through specific herbs and teas, and the role of key supplements and tonics in preventive health.

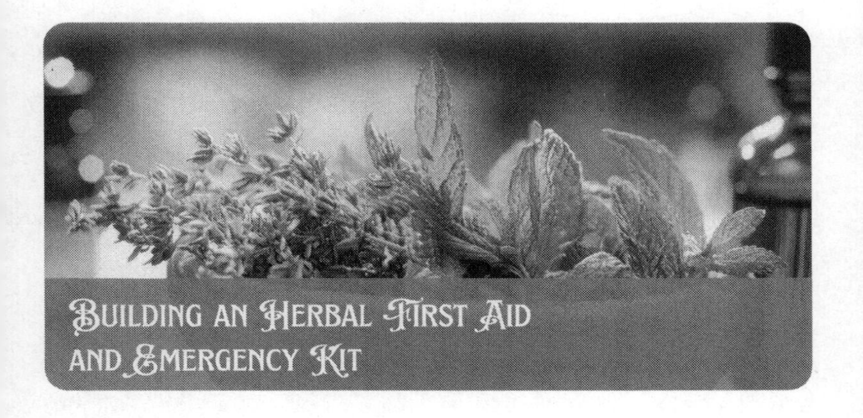

Building an Herbal First Aid and Emergency Kit

An herbal first aid and emergency kit serves as a valuable resource for treating common ailments and injuries at home. By preparing a kit stocked with essential herbs and remedies, you can be equipped to address minor health concerns and support your family's wellness needs.

When assembling your herbal first aid kit, start with a variety of herbal preparations that address common problems such as cuts, scrapes, burns, digestive upsets, and respiratory ailments. A good base for your kit is dried herbs that can be easily reconstituted into teas, tinctures, or poultices. Calendula, for example, is known for its potent healing properties and is ideal for treating minor cuts and scrapes. It can be used in an ointment or infused oil to promote healing and reduce inflammation. Similarly, comfrey, often called "knitbone," is excellent for promoting healing of broken bones and soft tissue injuries.

For digestive problems, add peppermint and ginger to your kit. Peppermint tea can soothe an upset stomach and relieve nausea, while ginger is known for its anti-inflammatory properties and ability to aid digestion. If you have ginger root or dried ginger on hand, you can make a soothing tea for digestive upset.

For respiratory problems, herbs such as mullein and thyme can be beneficial. Mullein can be made into a tea or infusion to soothe coughs and promote lung health, while thyme can be used to make a potent syrup for cough relief. Both herbs have antimicrobial properties, making them effective choices for supporting respiratory health.

In addition to dried herbs, include essential oils such as tea tree and lavender in your kit. Tea tree oil is a powerful antiseptic that can be applied topically to prevent infection in minor wounds, while lavender oil is known for its calming effects and can help reduce anxiety or promote sleep. Remember to dilute essential oils in a carrier oil before applying them to the skin.

An herbal first-aid kit should also include a variety of ready-to-use preparations, such as herbal ointments, salves, or tinctures. These can provide immediate relief when needed. For example, a soothing herbal ointment made from marigold, comfrey, and beeswax can be invaluable for treating minor burns or skin irritations.

To ensure that your herbal first aid kit is effective and safe, review and update its contents regularly. Check expiration dates on tinctures and ointments and replenish any used items. Familiarize yourself with the herbs and their uses so you can respond quickly and confidently in an emergency.

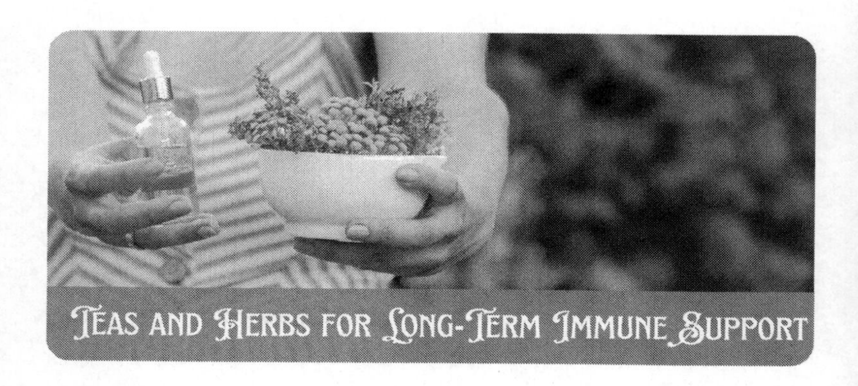

Teas and Herbs for Long-Term Immune Support

A robust immune system is essential for long-term health and well-being. Incorporating certain teas and herbs into your daily routine can provide ongoing support for immune function, helping to prevent illness and maintain overall vitality.

When considering herbs for immune support, echinacea is often a first choice due to its reputation for enhancing the immune response. It has been shown to reduce the duration and severity of colds and respiratory infections. Incorporating echinacea tea into your routine during the colder months can help prepare your body to fight off seasonal illnesses. Drinking this tea regularly can also encourage the body's natural defenses to be on high alert, ready to fight off pathogens.

Another valuable immune support herb is Astragalus. Known for its adaptogenic properties, astragalus root helps strengthen the immune system and supports the body's response to stress. It can be enjoyed as a tea or taken in capsule form. Adding Astragalus to soups or broths can enhance flavor while providing health benefits. Regular consumption of this herb is especially beneficial for those experiencing chronic stress, as it helps the body maintain balance.

For those looking to incorporate more citrus into their wellness routine, the use of elderberry is highly effective. Elderberry syrup is known for its antiviral properties, making it an excellent choice for supporting immune health, especially during cold and flu season. Elderberry can be consumed in syrup form, added to teas, or taken as a supplement. Its rich antioxidant content, coupled with its ability to fight viral infections, makes it a staple in many homes.

In addition to these specific herbs, consider creating herbal blends for teas that support long-term immune health. A blend of ginger, lemon balm, and green tea can create a refreshing beverage that offers both flavor and immune support. Ginger adds warmth and anti-inflammatory properties, while lemon balm is known for its calming effects and ability to reduce stress. Green tea, rich in antioxidants, complements this blend by promoting overall health.

Consistency is key when taking herbs for immune support. By incorporating these teas and herbs into your daily routine, your body can benefit from their protective properties over time. Whether enjoyed as a warm cup of tea in the morning or a refreshing iced beverage in the afternoon, these immune-boosting herbs can become an integral part of your lifestyle.

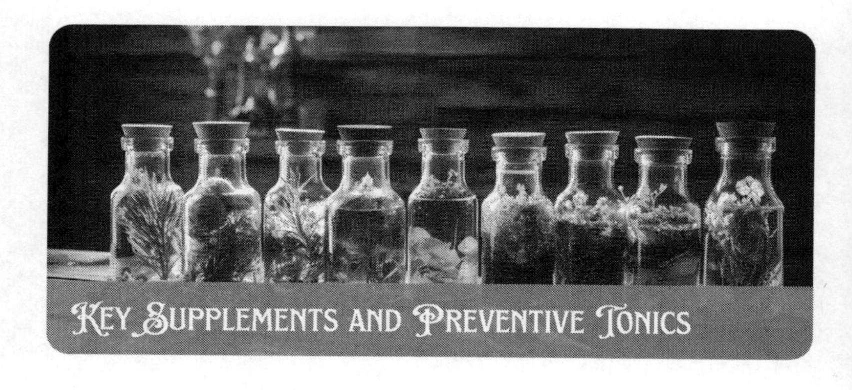

Key Supplements and Preventive Tonics

In addition to herbs and teas, certain supplements and tonics can play an important role in preventive health practices. These products can complement your herbal regimen and enhance your overall well-being, especially during times when your immune system needs extra support.

Vitamin C is one of the best known immune support supplements. It plays a vital role in several cellular functions of the immune system and has been shown to improve immune cell function. Regular intake of vitamin C, either through supplements or through foods rich in this vitamin, such as oranges, strawberries, and bell peppers, can help maintain a strong immune response.

Zinc is another important mineral that supports immune function. It is essential for the development and activation of T lymphocytes, which are critical for the immune response. Including zinc-rich foods such as nuts, seeds, and legumes in your diet can help boost your body's defenses. Alternatively, a zinc supplement may be considered, especially during cold and flu season.

Probiotics also play an important role in supporting immune health. They help maintain a balanced gut microbiome, which is critical for a healthy immune system. Regular consumption of fermented foods such as yogurt, kefir, sauerkraut, and kimchi can provide your body with beneficial bacteria that support digestive health and immunity. In addition, high-quality probiotic supplements can be taken to improve gut flora, especially during and after antibiotic treatment.

Preventive tonics made from herbs and natural ingredients can further support immune health. For example, a daily tonic made with apple cider vinegar, honey, and garlic can boost your immune system while supporting digestion. Apple cider vinegar has antimicrobial properties, honey is known for its soothing effects and nutritional benefits, and garlic is a powerful immune booster. Mixing these ingredients into a tonic can be a powerful addition to your daily routine, helping to prepare your body for potential illness.

Turmeric is another powerful ingredient to consider when creating preventative tonics. Known for its anti-inflammatory and antioxidant properties, turmeric can be added to smoothies, teas, or even taken as a supplement. Mixing turmeric with black pepper enhances its absorption, making it more effective in promoting overall health.

By incorporating these key supplements and preventative tonics into your daily regimen, you can strengthen your immune system and support your body's ability to fight off illness. Adopting a holistic approach to health that combines herbs, proper nutrition, and mindful practices will empower you to maintain long-term wellness and vitality. This proactive mindset not only improves your overall health, but also fosters a lifestyle that prioritizes prevention and self-care.

CHAPTER 3

Seasonal Cleansing and Detox Protocols

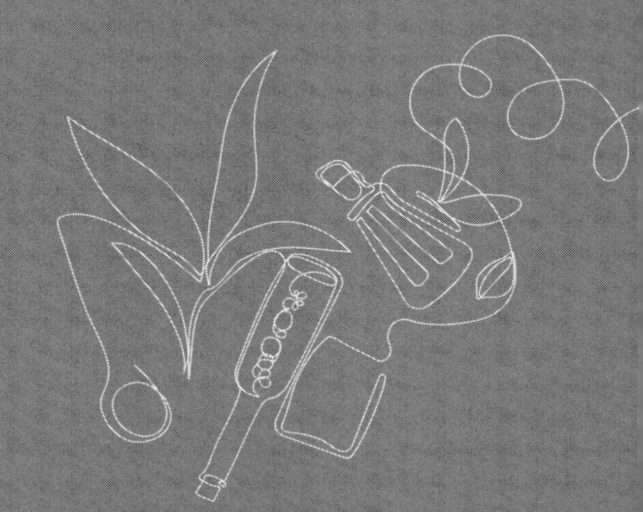

As the seasons change, so do the needs of our bodies. Seasonal cleansing and detoxification protocols provide an opportunity to reset, rejuvenate, and support our overall health. These practices not only help eliminate accumulated toxins, but also promote vitality and well-being. This chapter explores the importance of seasonal detoxification and offers insights into detox teas, simple cleanse schedules, detailed recipes for a 7-day herbal cleanse, and daily habits that support ongoing cleansing.

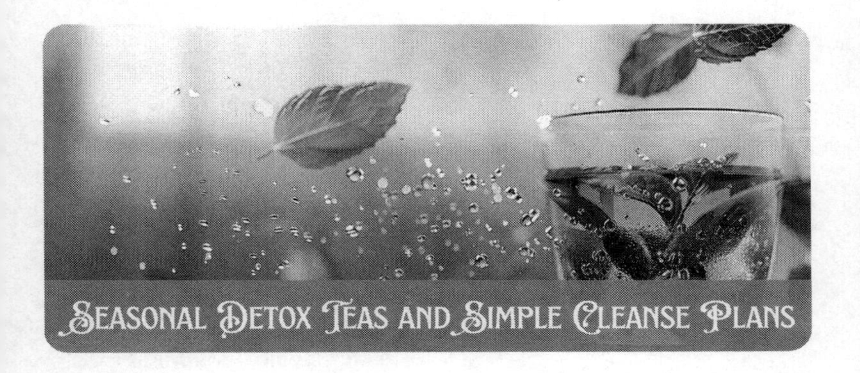

Seasonal Detox Teas and Simple Cleanse Plans

Herbal teas are a gentle and effective way to support the body's natural detoxification processes. Each season brings unique herbs that align with the body's needs, allowing you to tailor your cleansing regimen accordingly. In spring, for example, the body often craves rejuvenation after the long winter months. This is a great time to incorporate detox teas that focus on liver and gallbladder support. Dandelion root and milk thistle are great choices. Dandelion root aids digestion and stimulates bile production, while milk thistle protects the liver and supports its detoxification functions. An easy spring detox tea can be made by steeping dried dandelion root and milk thistle seeds in hot water, allowing the mixture to steep for about 10 minutes before straining and enjoying.

As summer approaches, it's important to support the body's ability to eliminate toxins with hydration and refreshing herbs. Herbal teas infused with hibiscus and peppermint are not only delicious, but also help cleanse the system. Hibiscus has diuretic properties that can help flush out toxins, while peppermint aids digestion and soothes the stomach. Brew a refreshing iced hibiscus tea and add a few sprigs of fresh peppermint for an invigorating drink that promotes detoxification and hydrates the body during hot weather.

In the fall, as the body prepares for the cooler months, it's beneficial to focus on warming teas that aid digestion and strengthen the immune system. Ginger and cinnamon are excellent additions for their warming properties and ability to stimulate circulation. A cozy blend of ginger tea infused with cinnamon and a splash of apple cider vinegar can provide warmth and comfort while promoting a healthy metabolism. This tea not only supports detoxification, but also helps ward off seasonal illnesses.

Winter is often a time for reflection and nurturing the body through cleansing. Root vegetables and warming herbs such as burdock root and licorice can be beneficial during this time. Burdock root is known for its blood-cleansing properties and can be steeped in a tea to support the kidneys and liver. Licorice root adds a naturally sweet flavor while helping to calm the gastrointestinal tract. Combining these herbs in a warm infusion can provide comfort and support during the colder months, making it an ideal winter detox tea.

In addition to herbal teas, simple cleansing regimens can help integrate detoxification into your seasonal routine. Consider setting aside one day each season to focus on cleansing. This could include eating mostly plant-based foods, drinking detox teas throughout the day, and prioritizing hydration. Eating seasonal produce not only provides nutrients, but also supports the body's natural detoxification processes. Incorporating seasonal foods such as leafy greens in the spring, berries in the summer, squash in the fall, and root vegetables in the winter can enhance your cleansing while connecting you to the rhythms of nature.

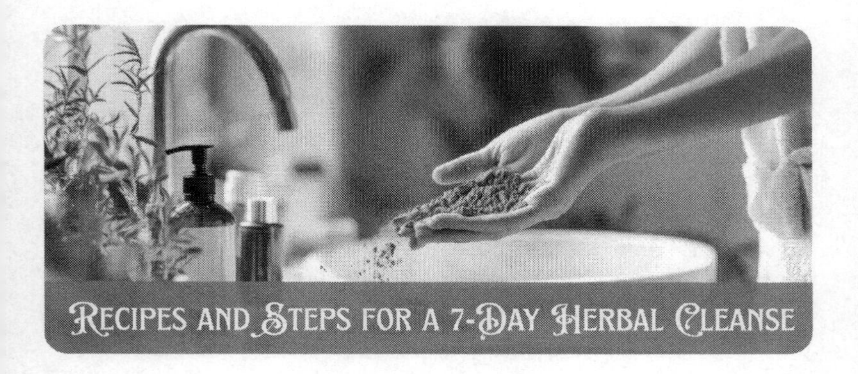

Recipes and Steps for a 7-Day Herbal Cleanse

Embarking on a 7-day herbal cleanse is a powerful way to rejuvenate your body and improve your overall health. This protocol involves consuming specific herbs, teas, and foods designed to support detoxification and promote a sense of well-being. The following is a simple yet effective plan for a week-long cleanse.

Day 1: Preparation and Intent Setting.

Begin your cleanse by setting clear intentions and preparing your body. This is a day of mental and physical preparation. Start with a light meal of fruits and vegetables. Start the day with a glass of warm lemon water to aid digestion. For tea, brew a cup of dandelion tea to support liver health. Reflect on your intentions for the cleanse, focusing on what you hope to accomplish in the coming week.

Days 2 to 4: The Detox Phase

During these days, prioritize consuming a variety of detoxifying herbal teas and nutrient-dense foods. Aim for at least three cups of herbal tea daily, alternating between dandelion, ginger, and nettle tea. Each of these teas has unique detoxifying properties. Dandelion tea aids liver function, ginger stimulates digestion, and nettle is packed with vitamins and minerals that support overall health.

For meals, focus on whole foods, emphasizing fruits, vegetables, whole grains, and legumes. Consider incorporating recipes like a quinoa salad with chopped kale, cucumbers, and a lemon tahini dressing, or a vegetable stir-fry with brown rice and fresh herbs.

Days 5 to 6: Herbal Support and Reflection

As you enter the second half of the cleanse, consider adding herbal supplements or tinctures to support your detoxification efforts. Milk thistle and burdock root capsules can be taken daily to support liver and kidney function. Continue your tea regimen and introduce a gentle detox smoothie made with spinach, banana, almond milk, and a scoop of spirulina to nourish your body.

Take time to reflect on how you are feeling physically and emotionally. Journaling your experience can help solidify the benefits and insights gained during this cleansing process.

Day 7: Gradual Reintroduction

The final day of your cleanse should focus on gradually reintroducing solid foods. Start the day with a soothing herbal tea, followed by a light breakfast such as oatmeal with fresh berries and a drizzle of honey. Continue drinking herbal teas and incorporating more complex meals throughout the day to allow your body to adjust.

Throughout the 7-day cleanse, it's important to prioritize hydration by drinking plenty of water. Consider adding a slice of lemon or cucumber to your water for an added refreshing twist.

This week-long herbal cleanse can serve as a powerful reset for your body, allowing you to eliminate toxins and reconnect with your health goals. By combining herbal teas, nourishing foods, and intentional reflection, you will cultivate a deeper understanding of your body's needs and support its natural ability to heal.

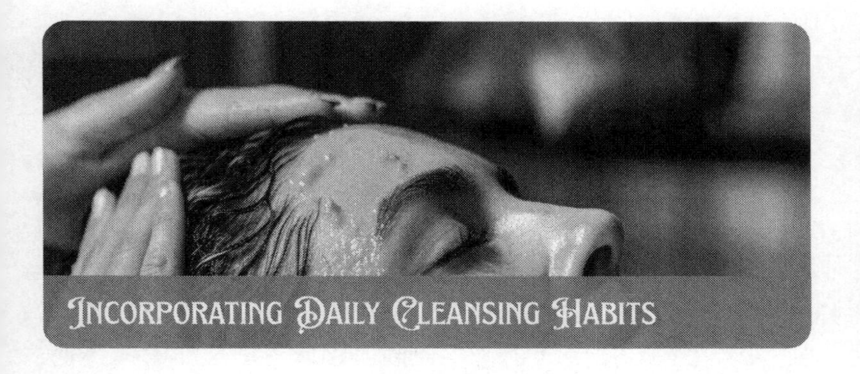

Incorporating Daily Cleansing Habits

Establishing daily cleansing habits can significantly improve your well-being and support your body's natural detoxification processes. These habits, when woven into your daily routine, promote a healthier lifestyle that emphasizes prevention and self-care.

Start by incorporating warm lemon water into your morning routine. This simple yet effective practice not only hydrates, but also aids in digestion and stimulates liver function. Adding a pinch of cayenne pepper can further enhance the detoxifying properties of the drink. This refreshing drink will help kickstart your metabolism and prepare your body for the day ahead.

Another valuable daily habit is to make sure you get enough fiber-rich foods. Incorporating fruits, vegetables, legumes, and whole grains into your meals not only supports healthy digestion, but also aids in the elimination of toxins. Fiber plays a crucial role in binding waste products in the digestive tract and promoting regular bowel movements. Consider starting your day with a fiber-rich breakfast, such as oatmeal topped with chia seeds and fresh fruit, to help keep your digestive system functioning optimally.

In addition to dietary choices, regular physical activity supports detoxification by increasing circulation and promoting sweating, both of which are essential for releasing toxins. Whether it's through yoga, walking, or more vigorous exercise, aim to incorporate movement into your daily routine. Practices such as yoga can also incorporate cleansing breathing techniques, such as pranayama, to further enhance detoxification.

Mindfulness and stress-reduction practices are also important for supporting the body's natural cleansing processes. Chronic stress can interfere with the body's ability to detoxify, leading to a buildup of toxins. Incorporating meditation, deep breathing exercises, or even simple moments of quiet reflection into your day can help manage stress levels. Consider setting aside a few minutes each day to engage in a mindfulness practice, which can help you center yourself and reduce tension.

Finally, get into the habit of drinking herbal teas daily. Choose a variety of detoxifying herbs, such as nettle, milk thistle, or ginger, and rotate them throughout the week. Each tea offers unique benefits and contributes to your overall cleansing goals. Enjoying a cup of herbal tea can serve as a moment of self-care and provide a comforting ritual to your day.

By incorporating these daily cleansing habits into your life, you create a sustainable approach to health and wellness that promotes detoxification and overall vitality. The key is consistency-prioritizing these habits will help you support your body's natural processes and cultivate a lifestyle that promotes balance and well-being.

CHAPTER 4

Herbal Practices for Enhanced Longevity and Vitality

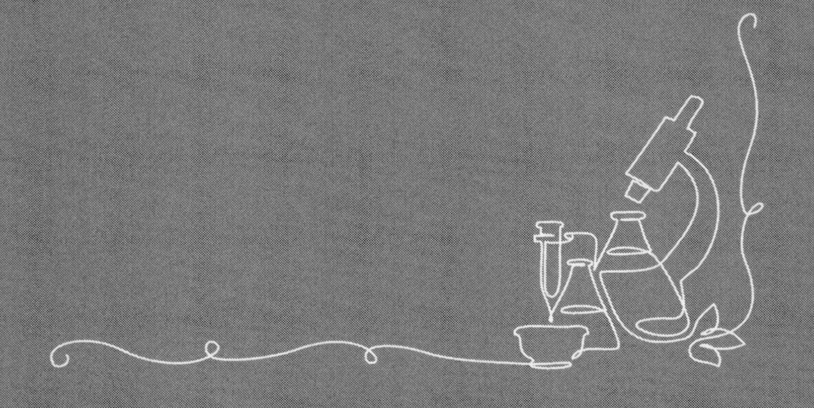

In the quest for longevity and vitality, herbal practices can play a pivotal role in supporting health as we age. As the body undergoes various changes, incorporating specific herbs and natural remedies into our daily routines can help maintain optimal health, improve resilience, and enhance overall well-being. This chapter explores herbal practices designed to support aging and cellular health; maintain joint, bone, and muscle integrity; and utilize adaptogens for sustained vitality and resilience.

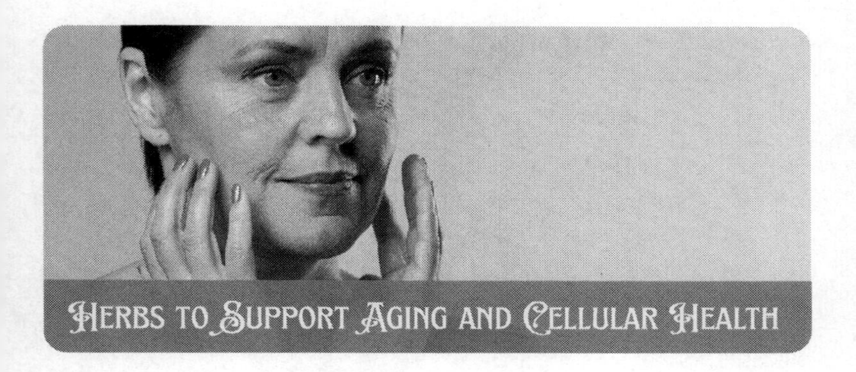

Herbs to Support Aging and Cellular Health

As we age, our bodies naturally undergo a myriad of changes that affect everything from cellular health to overall vitality. Incorporating certain herbs into our daily routines can help combat these age-related changes and promote longevity. One of the most celebrated herbs for supporting cellular health is turmeric, largely due to its active ingredient, curcumin.

Curcumin has potent antioxidant and anti-inflammatory properties that can combat oxidative stress - a major contributor to aging. Regularly incorporating turmeric into your diet, whether through teas, supplements, or culinary dishes, can help protect your cells and reduce the risk of age-related diseases.

Another powerful herb in the realm of aging is ashwagandha, an adaptogenic herb known for its ability to combat stress and promote overall wellness. Chronic stress can accelerate the aging process by increasing inflammation and negatively impacting mental health. Ashwagandha supports the body's stress response, helping to balance cortisol levels and improve resilience. Incorporating this herb into your routine can be as simple as taking it in powder form mixed into smoothies or as capsules.

Ginkgo biloba is another herb that has garnered attention for its potential benefits in improving cognitive function and circulation. By improving blood flow to the brain, ginkgo may help improve memory and cognitive performance, making it especially valuable for older adults. Consuming Ginkgo biloba in capsule or tea form can provide ongoing support for brain health.

In addition, the herb resveratrol, found in the skin of grapes and red wine, has gained popularity for its antioxidant properties and potential anti-aging effects.

Resveratrol is thought to promote longevity by activating certain genes associated with aging and cellular repair. While it can be obtained through diet by consuming red wine or grapes, high-quality resveratrol supplements can also provide concentrated benefits.

Maintaining cellular health also means making sure the body gets enough vitamins and minerals. Herbs such as nettle and alfalfa are rich in essential nutrients such as vitamins A, C, and K, as well as minerals such as calcium and magnesium. These herbs can be enjoyed in the form of teas or capsules, contributing to overall health while providing the body with the nutrients it needs to function optimally as it ages.

By embracing these herbs and incorporating them into daily routines, individuals can take proactive steps to support their health and longevity. This holistic approach empowers one to not only age gracefully, but to maintain a vibrant and active lifestyle well into later years.

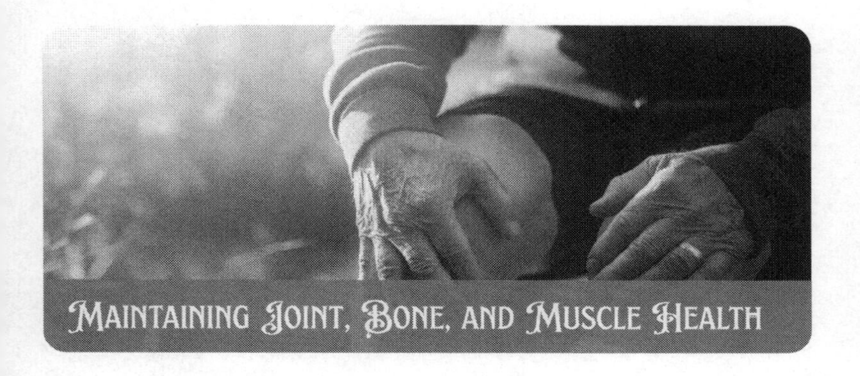

Maintaining Joint, Bone, and Muscle Health

As we age, joint, bone, and muscle health becomes increasingly important for maintaining mobility and overall quality of life. Integrating certain herbs and dietary practices can support these areas, helping to prevent discomfort and promote longevity.

One of the most widely used herbs for joint health is turmeric. The curcumin in turmeric has anti-inflammatory properties that can reduce the pain and swelling associated with arthritis and joint discomfort.

Consuming turmeric in the form of a warm tea or adding it to meals can provide relief for those experiencing joint problems. In addition, ginger is another powerful anti-inflammatory herb that can help manage joint pain and stiffness. A daily ginger tea or fresh ginger added to smoothies can serve as a powerful joint health remedy.

Boswellia, also known as Indian incense, has gained attention for its ability to reduce inflammation and pain in the joints. Boswellia extracts have shown promise in studies related to osteoarthritis and rheumatoid arthritis, helping to improve joint function and reduce discomfort. Taking boswellia as a supplement or extract can provide targeted support for joint health.

To maintain bone strength, it is important to include herbs rich in calcium and vitamin K. Nettle and alfalfa are excellent sources of these nutrients and can be enjoyed as teas or incorporated into meals.

In addition, horsetail is a lesser-known herb that is high in silica, which is essential for bone formation and maintenance. Horsetail can be taken as a tea or supplement to effectively support bone health.

Maintaining muscle health is also a critical component of overall vitality as we age. Regular physical activity combined with herbal support can help maintain muscle mass and strength. Incorporating adaptogenic herbs such as Rhodiola rosea can improve physical performance and reduce fatigue, making exercise more enjoyable and sustainable. Rhodiola has been shown to improve stamina and endurance, supporting muscle health during physical activity.

In addition, maintaining adequate hydration and nutrition is critical for joint and muscle health. Drinking herbal teas that support hydration, such as hibiscus or peppermint, can promote overall wellness. These herbs not only provide hydration, but also offer additional health benefits that help maintain muscle and joint function.

By taking a holistic approach to maintaining joint, bone, and muscle health, individuals can actively support their bodies as they age. Incorporating these herbs and practices into daily routines promotes a sense of well-being and resilience, ensuring that one can continue to enjoy an active and fulfilling lifestyle.

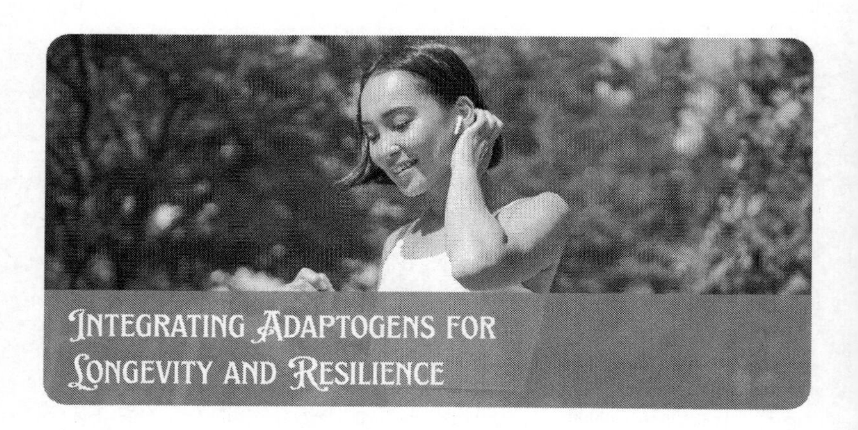

Integrating Adaptogens for Longevity and Resilience

Adaptogens are a unique class of herbs that help the body adapt to stressors and promote overall balance and resilience. As we navigate the complexities of modern life, incorporating adaptogens into our daily routines can provide significant benefits for longevity and well-being. These herbs support the body's stress response, increase energy levels, and contribute to overall vitality.

One of the most well-known adaptogens is ashwagandha, which has been used in traditional Ayurvedic medicine for centuries.

Ashwagandha helps lower cortisol levels, the hormone associated with stress, and promotes a sense of calm and balance. Regular use of ashwagandha can lead to improved mood, increased focus, and increased energy levels, making it an invaluable addition to any wellness routine. It can be taken as a powder, mixed into smoothies, taken in capsules, or even brewed into a warm tea.

Another potent adaptogen is holy basil, or tulsi, which is known for its ability to reduce stress and support immune function. Holy basil contains compounds that help regulate cortisol levels and support the body's natural response to stress. Incorporating holy basil into your daily routine can be as simple as drinking a cup of holy basil tea or using the dried leaves in cooking. Its uplifting scent and flavor make it a delightful way to enhance daily wellness.

Rhodiola rosea is also gaining recognition for its energizing properties and ability to enhance mental performance. It can help combat fatigue, improve stamina, and support cognitive function. Rhodiola is particularly beneficial for those experiencing chronic stress or fatigue, as it can help the body adapt to physical and emotional challenges. Incorporating Rhodiola into your routine as a supplement or tea can provide the necessary support for resilience and longevity.

To fully reap the benefits of adaptogens, consider creating a daily ritual that includes these herbs. For example, starting the day with an adaptogen smoothie that includes ashwagandha or a warm cup of holy basil tea can set a positive tone for the day.

Throughout the day, you can also enjoy adaptogen-infused snacks or tonics for sustained energy and balance.

In addition to these specific adaptogens, a balanced diet rich in whole foods, regular exercise, and mindfulness practices can amplify their effects. Engaging in stress-reduction techniques such as yoga, meditation, or deep-breathing exercises can enhance the body's ability to manage stress and support overall health.

By incorporating adaptogens into your daily routine, you empower your body to meet life's challenges with grace and resilience. These powerful herbs not only contribute to longevity, but also promote a holistic approach to well-being, ensuring that you can thrive in mind and body as you age. Incorporating adaptogens into your daily practice cultivates a deeper connection to your health and a proactive approach to maintaining vitality throughout the years.

CHAPTER 5

Building Resilience to Stress and Enhancing Sleep Quality

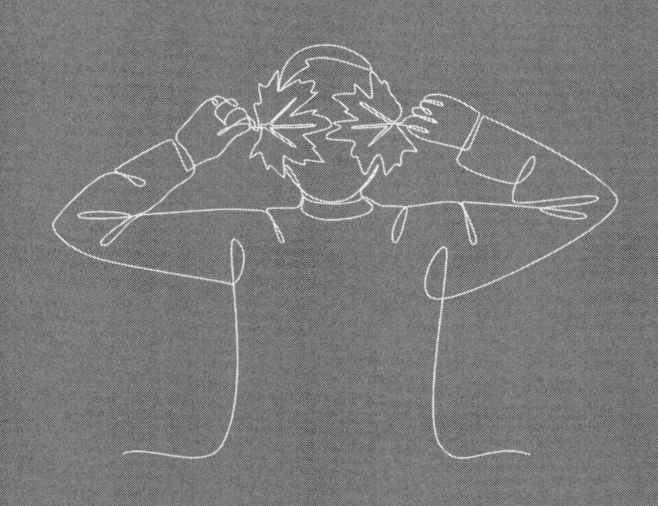

Managing stress and ensuring restful sleep are critical components of maintaining overall health and well-being in today's fast-paced world. The body's ability to cope with stress directly affects physical health, emotional balance, and sleep quality.

This chapter examines effective herbs and techniques for reducing stress, outlines rituals and blends that promote better sleep, and explores natural remedies that combat fatigue and overwhelm. By adopting these practices, individuals can cultivate resilience to life's pressures and create an environment conducive to deep, restorative sleep.

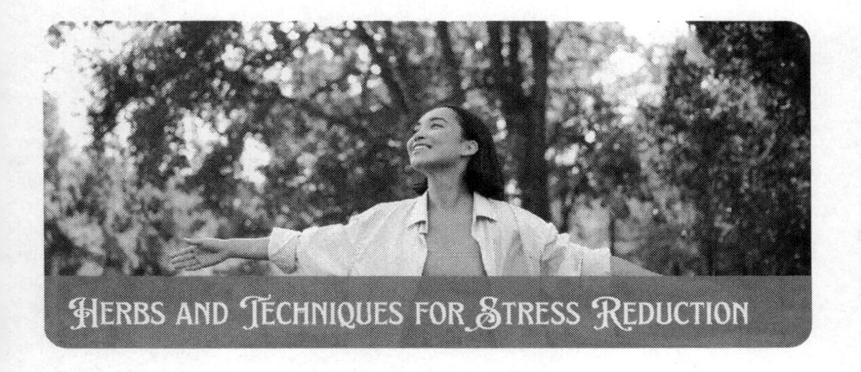

Herbs and Techniques for Stress Reduction

Stress is an inevitable part of life, but how we respond to it can have a profound effect on our health. Incorporating herbal remedies into your daily routine can provide powerful support for managing stress and promoting relaxation.

One of the most well-known herbs for stress relief is ashwagandha, an adaptogen that helps the body adapt to stressors and balance cortisol levels. This herb is known for its calming properties and has been shown to improve mood and reduce anxiety. Incorporating ashwagandha into your regimen can be as simple as taking it in capsule form, adding the powder to smoothies, or brewing a calming tea.

Another effective herb for reducing stress is lavender. Known for its calming aroma, lavender can help relieve tension and anxiety. It can be used in several forms, including essential oil for aromatherapy, dried flowers for tea, or even infused into bath products. A warm cup of lavender tea before bed can not only help reduce stress, but also prepare the mind and body for a restful night's sleep. In addition, chamomile tea is a wonderful choice for relaxation, as it has mild sedative effects that can help calm the nervous system and promote a sense of calm.

Incorporating mindfulness and relaxation techniques along with herbal remedies can enhance their effects. Practices such as yoga, meditation, and deep breathing exercises can significantly reduce stress levels. Practicing yoga not only encourages physical movement, but also promotes mindfulness, allowing individuals to reconnect with their bodies and release tension.

A few minutes of focused breathing, such as inhaling deeply to the count of four, holding for four, and exhaling to the count of four, can immediately reduce stress levels and create a sense of calm.

Regular exercise is another effective way to manage stress. Exercise releases endorphins, which are natural mood enhancers that can counteract feelings of stress and anxiety. Whether it's a brisk walk, a dance class, or a more structured workout, finding enjoyable ways to incorporate movement into your day can help maintain emotional balance.

Ultimately, the key to stress reduction is finding a combination of herbal support and lifestyle practices that resonate with you. By developing a personalized approach to stress management, individuals can build resilience, improve overall well-being, and foster a sense of calm in the midst of life's challenges.

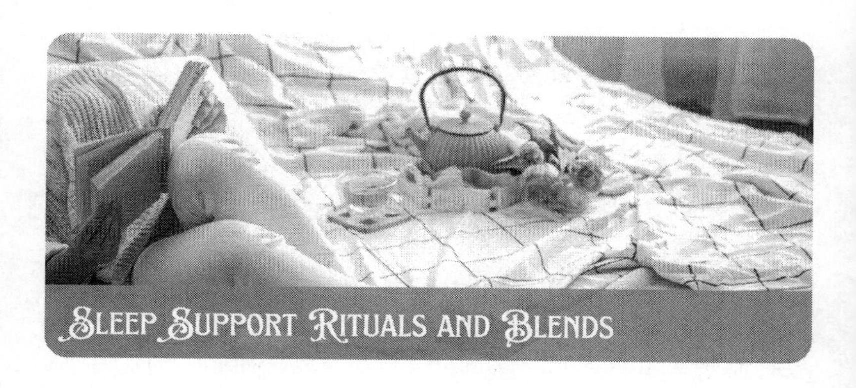

Sleep Support Rituals and Blends

Quality sleep is essential for physical health, emotional well-being, and cognitive function. Creating a calming bedtime routine that includes herbal support can help signal your body that it's time to wind down and prepare for restorative sleep. Establishing a consistent sleep schedule, where you go to bed and wake up at the same time each day, can help regulate your body's internal clock and improve overall sleep quality.

Incorporating herbal teas into your nighttime routine can be a gentle way to promote relaxation. Herbs such as valerian root, passionflower, and lemon balm are known for their sleep-supporting properties. Valerian root has been used for centuries to treat insomnia and is particularly effective at reducing the time it takes to fall asleep.

A warm cup of valerian tea, perhaps combined with chamomile for added sedation, can create a soothing evening ritual. Passion flower is another wonderful sleep herb, known for its ability to reduce anxiety and promote deeper sleep. Drinking a tea made from dried passionflower leaves can help calm the mind and ease the transition to sleep.

Creating a nighttime ritual that incorporates aromatherapy can further promote relaxation. Diffusing calming essential oils such as lavender, bergamot, or cedarwood in your bedroom can create a serene atmosphere conducive to sleep. You might also consider using a sleep pillow spray containing these essential oils and lightly misting your pillow before bed. This sensory experience reinforces the connection between scent and sleep, signaling to your body that it's time to relax.

Engaging in calming activities before bedtime, such as reading, journaling, or practicing gentle stretches, can also be beneficial. These practices help the mind transition away from the stresses of the day and promote a sense of peace. Establishing at least 30 minutes of unwinding before bed, free from screens and stimulating activities, can greatly improve your ability to fall asleep and stay asleep.

In addition, creating a restful sleep environment is essential for quality rest. Make sure your bedroom is dark, cool, and quiet, and minimize distractions that can disrupt sleep. Investing in blackout curtains, white noise machines, or comfortable bedding can significantly improve your sleep quality.

By adopting these sleep-supporting rituals and herbal blends, individuals can cultivate an environment that promotes relaxation and restful sleep, allowing the body and mind to rejuvenate and recover during the night.

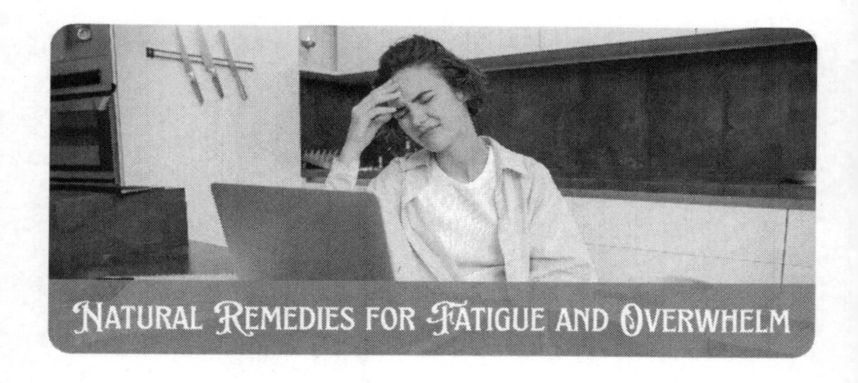

Natural Remedies for Fatigue and Overwhelm

Fatigue and feelings of being overwhelmed can be debilitating, affecting daily life and overall well-being. Incorporating natural remedies into your routine can provide relief and support for both physical and emotional exhaustion. One effective approach is to harness the power of adaptogenic herbs, which help the body adapt to stress and increase energy levels.

Rhodiola rosea is an adaptogen known for its ability to combat fatigue and increase stamina. It works by regulating the body's stress response and reducing cortisol levels. Regular use of Rhodiola can help improve mental performance and physical stamina. This herb can be taken in capsule form, added to smoothies, or brewed into a tea for daily support.

Another excellent remedy for fatigue is the use of ginseng, specifically Asian ginseng (Panax ginseng) or American ginseng (Panax quinquefolius). Both varieties are celebrated for their energizing properties and ability to enhance physical performance and cognitive function. Ginseng can be consumed in the form of tea, tincture, or capsules. Incorporating ginseng into your daily routine can help boost your energy levels and combat feelings of fatigue.

Nourishing the body with nutrient-dense foods is also crucial in combating fatigue. Include whole foods that are rich in vitamins and minerals, such as leafy greens, nuts, seeds, and whole grains. Iron-rich foods, such as spinach and lentils, can help prevent fatigue caused by iron deficiency, while complex carbohydrates provide sustained energy throughout the day.

Hydration also plays an important role in fighting fatigue. Dehydration can lead to feelings of lethargy and exhaustion, so it's important to drink plenty of water throughout the day. Herbal teas can also help with hydration while providing additional health benefits. Herbal infusions of nettle or peppermint can invigorate and refresh while supporting overall well-being.

In addition to herbal remedies, coping with overwhelm requires the use of effective stress management techniques. Practicing mindfulness meditation can help center the mind and reduce feelings of anxiety and stress. Taking a few minutes each day to engage in deep breathing exercises or guided meditation can bring clarity and calm, allowing you to face daily challenges with greater ease.

By incorporating these natural remedies for fatigue and overwhelm, individuals can cultivate resilience and foster a greater sense of vitality. A holistic approach that combines adaptogens, nutritious foods, and mindful practices can create a powerful framework for combating fatigue and enhancing overall well-being. This proactive strategy enables individuals to navigate life's demands with energy and purpose, ensuring that they can fully engage with the world around them.

CHAPTER 6

Supporting Family Health with Herbal Practices

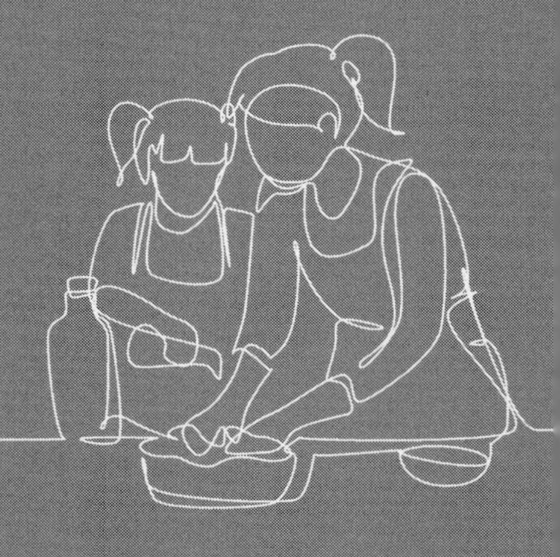

The health and well-being of a family is often intertwined, with each member's wellness impacting the others. Integrating herbal practices into family routines can promote a culture of health and self-care that benefits everyone.

This chapter focuses on how to customize herbal routines for each family member, explore safe herbs for children and elderly adults, and implement family-strengthening immune protocols. By adopting these practices, families can cultivate resilience, enhance vitality, and foster a supportive environment for health and healing.

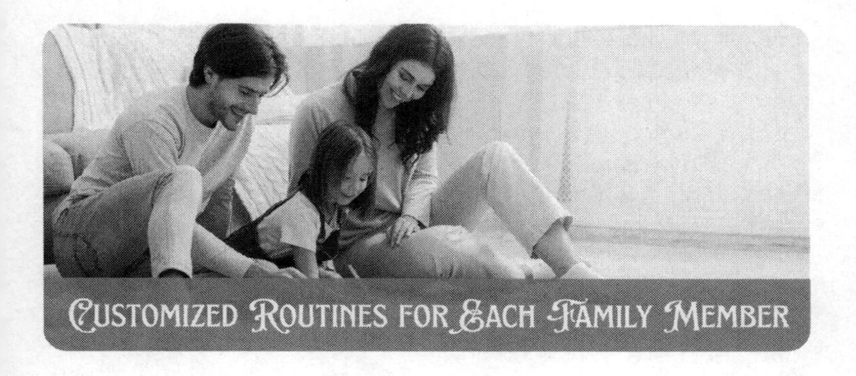

Customized Routines for Each Family Member

Creating personalized herbal routines for each family member is essential to addressing individual health needs while promoting wellness within the family unit. Each person has unique health challenges and needs based on age, lifestyle, and specific health concerns. Tailoring herbal practices to these needs not only enhances the effectiveness of the remedies, but also encourages each family member to become actively involved in their health journey.

For children, the focus should be on gentle yet effective herbs that support growth, immunity, and overall health. Herbal teas made with chamomile or lemon balm can be soothing for anxious children and help them relax before bedtime. In addition, adding elderberry syrup to their routine can provide a natural boost to their immune system, especially during cold and flu season. Known for its antiviral properties, elderberry is a delicious way to support children's health.

For teens, addressing the unique challenges of adolescence is key. Herbs such as stinging nettle and red clover can support hormonal balance, while peppermint tea can help with digestion, especially during the stressful school year. Encouraging teens to make their own herbal teas or smoothies can foster a sense of independence and personal responsibility for their health.

For adults, the focus may shift to stress management and maintaining energy levels. Adaptogens such as ashwagandha and rhodiola can be incorporated into daily routines to help combat the stresses of work and family life. Simple routines could include morning smoothies enriched with these herbs or evening teas that promote relaxation, such as valerian or lemon balm.

For older family members, the importance of maintaining vitality and preventing chronic disease cannot be overstated. Herbal practices for seniors should focus on supporting joint health, digestion, and cognitive function. Incorporating turmeric and ginger into meals can help manage inflammation, while ginkgo biloba may be beneficial for cognitive support. Regular consumption of herbal teas that emphasize these aspects can improve quality of life and promote a sense of well-being.

Each family member can benefit from a structured approach that includes regular health check-ins to assess how they are feeling and which herbs or routines work best for them. Creating a family health calendar can serve as a fun way to track herbal intake, share recipes, and remind everyone of their wellness goals. This practice promotes accountability and encourages open discussions about health within the family.

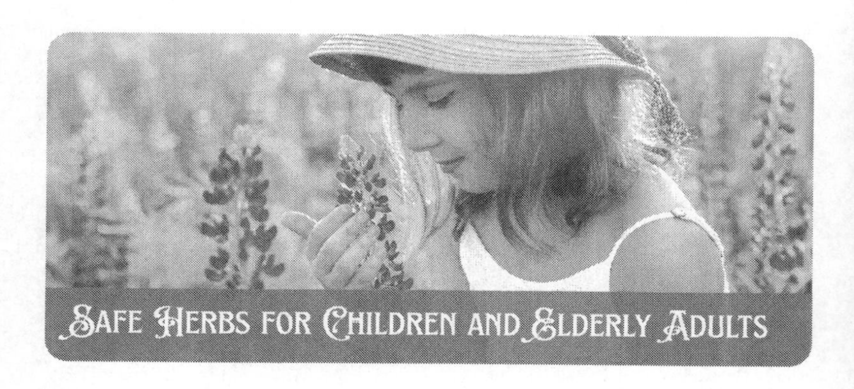

Safe Herbs for Children and Elderly Adults

When incorporating herbal practices into the health routines of children and elderly adults, safety is paramount. It is essential to choose herbs that are known for their gentle effects and minimal side effects. For children, age-appropriate dosing is critical, as their smaller body size requires careful consideration of herb potency and concentration.

Herbs such as chamomile and lemon balm are excellent choices for children. Chamomile, known for its calming properties, can help soothe upset stomachs and promote restful sleep. A mild chamomile tea can be easily prepared, making it a comforting evening ritual. Lemon balm also offers a gentle approach to reducing anxiety and stress in children, and it can be enjoyed as a refreshing tea or added to smoothies.

Elderberry is another safe and effective herb for children, particularly for its immune-boosting properties. Elderberry syrup can be a tasty addition to their diet, providing essential vitamins and antioxidants. It is important to choose high-quality, organic elderberry products to ensure safety and efficacy.

For elderly adults, many herbs can support their health while being mindful of potential interactions with medications. Ginger and turmeric are great options, known for their anti-inflammatory properties and ability to support joint health. Both herbs can be easily added to meals or taken as supplements, helping to alleviate discomfort associated with arthritis or other inflammatory conditions.

Another valuable herb for seniors is hawthorn, which can support heart health and circulation. Hawthorn berries can be taken as a tincture or in tea form, offering gentle support without significant side effects. Similarly, ginkgo biloba can help enhance cognitive function and improve memory, making it a beneficial addition to the health regimen of older adults.

When introducing new herbs to children or elderly adults, it's important to consult with a healthcare provider, particularly if there are pre-existing conditions or medications involved. Educating family members about the benefits and appropriate uses of these herbs can empower them to make informed choices about their health.

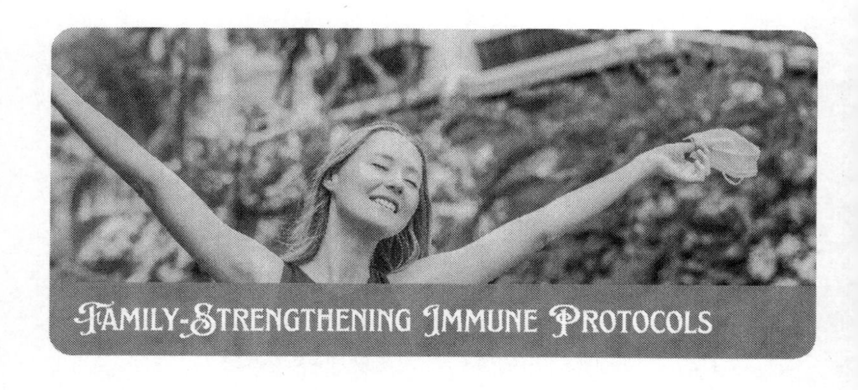

Family-Strengthening Immune Protocols

A strong immune system is essential for overall health, especially in families where different members may have different health challenges. Implementing family-strengthening immune protocols can help strengthen the body's defenses and promote overall wellness. These protocols can include dietary practices, herbal supplements, and lifestyle changes that strengthen the immune system.

One effective approach is to focus on a nutrient-dense diet rich in vitamins and minerals known for their immune-boosting properties. Foods high in vitamin C, such as citrus fruits, bell peppers, and leafy greens, can be highlighted in meals and snacks.

Garlic, with its antimicrobial properties, can also be incorporated into family meals to enhance flavor while boosting immunity. Encouraging family members to prepare meals together can promote a sense of unity and reinforce healthy eating habits.

Incorporating certain herbs into daily routines can also be beneficial. Echinacea, elderberry, or nettle herbal teas can be offered regularly, especially during cold and flu season. For younger family members, making herbal teas more appealing by adding honey or combining them with fruit can encourage them to participate in this immune support ritual. Adults may also benefit from taking herbal tinctures that boost immunity, such as astragalus or reishi mushroom extract, which can be easily added to smoothies or taken directly.

Regular physical activity is essential to maintaining a healthy immune system. Encouraging family outings that include exercise, such as hiking, biking, or family sports, can promote bonding while supporting physical health. Physical activity helps increase circulation, reduce stress, and improve overall well-being, all of which are important for immune function.

In addition to diet and lifestyle changes, incorporating relaxation techniques can help manage stress levels, which in turn supports immune health. Family mindfulness practices, such as yoga or meditation, can be a fun way to relax together while teaching valuable stress management skills. Setting aside a specific time each week for family relaxation sessions can create a routine that emphasizes the importance of mental and emotional well-being.

By establishing these family-strengthening immune protocols, families can work together to foster a culture of health that benefits every member. Incorporating these practices into daily life helps create an environment that prioritizes wellness and ensures that everyone feels supported and empowered in their health journey. By taking a proactive approach, families can cultivate resilience and vitality, improving their overall quality of life and well-being.

CHAPTER 7

Adapting to Modern Life with Ancient Herbal Wisdom

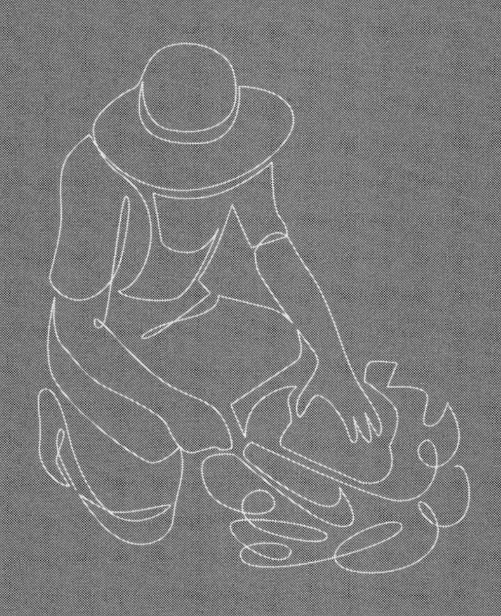

In an age of rapid change and constant demands, the search for balance and well-being has never been more important. Ancient herbal wisdom offers valuable insights and tools for navigating the complexities of modern life.

By integrating these time-honored practices into our daily routines, we can build resilience, improve our health, and reconnect with the natural world. This chapter explores how to find balance through herbal practices, use nature's pharmacy to combat environmental toxins, and implement daily habits that promote physical, mental, and emotional wellness.

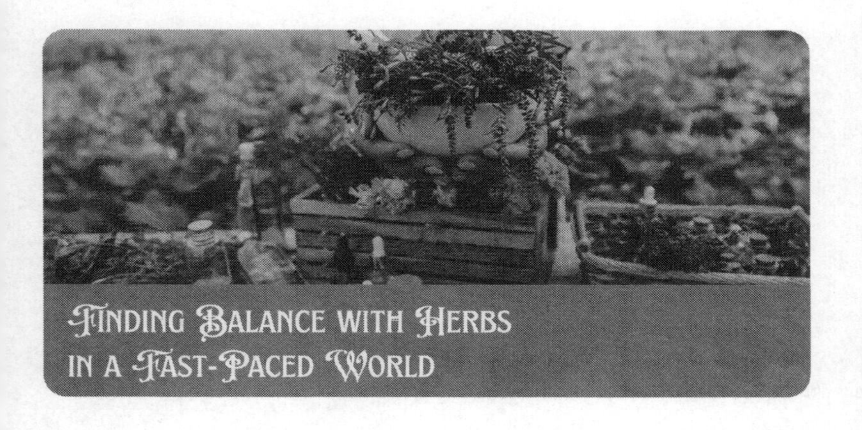

Finding Balance with Herbs in a Fast-Paced World

The fast-paced nature of modern life often leaves people feeling overwhelmed, disconnected, and tired. Finding balance in the midst of these challenges is essential to maintaining overall health and well-being. Herbs have been used for centuries to assist in this endeavor, offering natural solutions for stress management and emotional stability.

Adaptogens, a unique class of herbs, play an important role in helping individuals adapt to stressors while promoting balance within the body. Ashwagandha is one such adaptogen, known for its ability to lower cortisol levels and increase resilience to stress. Incorporating ashwagandha into your daily routine can be achieved through supplements, powders mixed into smoothies, or as an infusion in herbal teas. This gentle herb empowers the body to respond more effectively to stress, allowing individuals to regain a sense of calm and clarity.

Rhodiola rosea is another potent adaptogen that helps combat fatigue and supports mental clarity. By increasing the body's ability to cope with physical and emotional stress, Rhodiola can improve focus and energy levels. Taking Rhodiola in capsule form or as a tea can be an effective way to incorporate its benefits into a busy lifestyle, helping you maintain productivity while managing stress.

In addition to adaptogens, herbal teas can be an effective way to cultivate balance and relaxation throughout the day. Herbal blends containing chamomile, lemon balm, and peppermint offer calming properties that promote mental clarity and relaxation.

A calming tea ritual, especially in the afternoon or evening, can serve as a restorative practice that allows individuals to pause, reflect, and recalibrate in the midst of their busy schedules.

Establishing healthy routines that incorporate herbal practices can greatly enhance one's ability to find balance. Creating a morning ritual that includes herbal teas or supplements can set a positive tone for the day. Similarly, setting aside time in the evening for herbal baths or aromatherapy with essential oils such as lavender or bergamot can provide a soothing transition into the night.

By embracing the wisdom of herbs and making conscious choices, individuals can effectively adapt to the demands of modern life while maintaining their health and well-being. The key lies in recognizing the importance of self-care and integrating these ancient practices into daily routines to foster a harmonious relationship with oneself and the world.

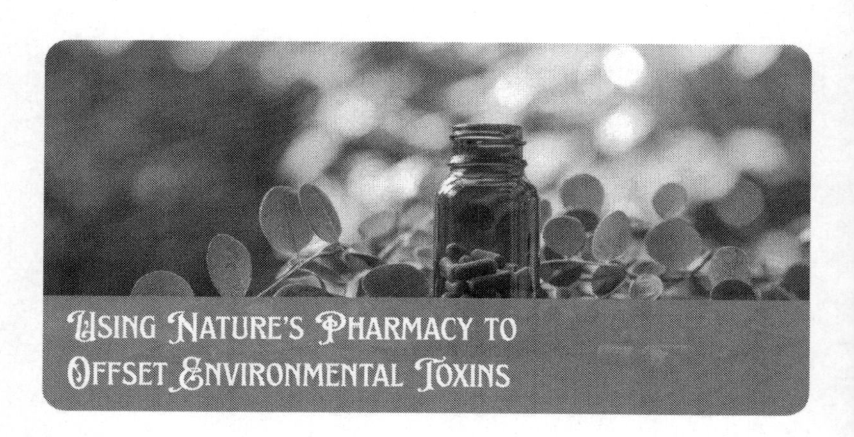

In our increasingly industrialized world, exposure to environmental toxins is a growing concern that can adversely affect health. These toxins can be found in the air we breathe, the food we eat, and even the products we use on a daily basis. Fortunately, nature offers a variety of herbs and plants that can help counteract the harmful effects of these environmental stressors, effectively serving as nature's pharmacy.

One of the most notable herbs for detoxification is milk thistle, which is known for its ability to protect the liver. The active ingredient silymarin helps neutralize toxins and promotes liver cell regeneration. Incorporating milk thistle into your regimen, whether through capsules, tinctures, or teas, can provide essential support for the liver and aid the body's natural detoxification processes.

Dandelion is another powerful ally in the fight against environmental toxins. Both the leaves and roots are beneficial for supporting liver function and promoting healthy digestion. Dandelion tea or tinctures can increase the body's ability to eliminate waste and toxins. In addition, dandelion acts as a diuretic, helping to flush out toxins through increased urine production.

The importance of antioxidants in combating environmental toxins cannot be overstated. Herbs such as turmeric and ginger are rich in antioxidants that help neutralize harmful free radicals in the body. Turmeric, with its active compound curcumin, has been extensively studied for its anti-inflammatory and antioxidant properties. Incorporating turmeric into meals, teas, or supplements can boost the body's defenses against oxidative stress.

In addition to these detoxifying herbs, a diet rich in fruits and vegetables can further support the body's ability to fight toxins. Foods such as cruciferous vegetables (broccoli, cauliflower, and kale) are known to contain liver-supporting compounds that enhance detoxification pathways. Leafy greens and berries are also packed with vitamins and minerals that contribute to overall health and resistance to environmental challenges.

Creating a home environment that minimizes exposure to toxins is also important. Using natural cleaning products, reducing plastic use, and incorporating air-purifying houseplants can help create a healthier living space. Herbs such as aloe vera and spider plants are excellent choices for improving indoor air quality and contributing to a healthier environment.

By harnessing the power of nature's pharmacy, individuals can take proactive steps to offset environmental toxins and improve their well-being. Embracing herbal remedies and dietary practices not only supports the body's detoxification processes, but also fosters a deeper connection to nature, promoting overall health in our modern world.

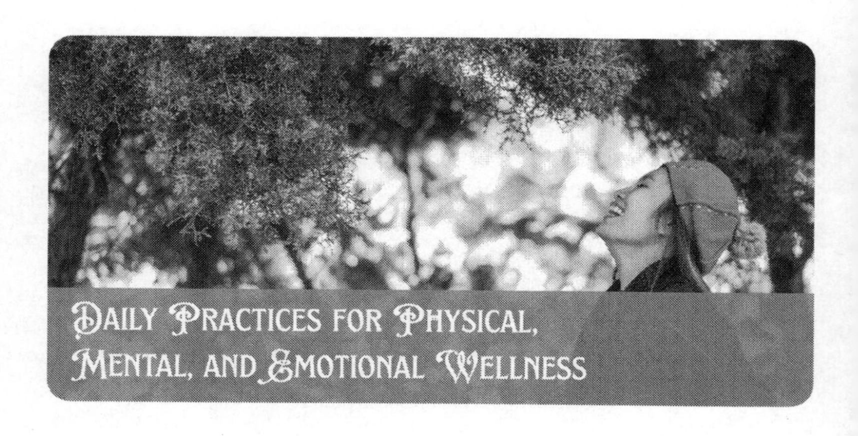

Daily Practices for Physical, Mental, and Emotional Wellness

Incorporating daily practices that support physical, mental, and emotional well-being is fundamental to achieving a balanced and healthy lifestyle. By intentionally weaving these practices into your routine, you can build resilience and improve your overall well-being.

Physical activity is a cornerstone of health and can take many forms, from brisk walking to yoga. Regular exercise not only strengthens the body, but also releases endorphins, which improve mood and reduce stress. Aim for at least 30 minutes of moderate physical activity most days of the week. Activities that you enjoy, such as dancing, biking, or hiking, can make this routine more enjoyable and sustainable.

Complementing physical activity with herbal support can enhance its benefits. Herbal teas that promote relaxation, such as chamomile or passionflower, can be incorporated into a post-exercise routine to provide a soothing end to a workout. These teas can help calm the mind and body, allowing you to transition smoothly into your day or evening.

Mental wellness is equally important and can be supported through mindfulness practices. Daily meditation, even for just a few minutes, can have a significant impact on mental clarity and emotional resilience.

Techniques such as guided visualization, breath awareness, or body scans can help center your thoughts and reduce anxiety. Incorporating herbal support, such as adaptogenic teas, can further enhance these practices and promote a sense of calm and focus.

Journaling is another powerful practice for promoting emotional wellness. Taking time each day to reflect on thoughts, feelings, and experiences can provide clarity and promote emotional processing. Herbal teas such as lemon balm or rose can create a calming atmosphere while journaling, promoting relaxation and emotional expression.

Diet also plays an important role in supporting overall wellness. A balanced diet rich in whole foods, including fruits, vegetables, whole grains, and healthy fats, provides the body with the essential nutrients it needs to function optimally. Herbs such as basil, oregano, and thyme not only add flavor, but also offer health benefits. Regularly incorporating these herbs into meals can aid digestion and contribute to overall health.

Finally, ensuring adequate hydration is a simple yet powerful practice. Drinking water infused with herbs such as mint or citrus throughout the day can help maintain hydration levels and support metabolic functions. Herbal infusions can also be enjoyed, providing additional health benefits while nourishing the body.

By incorporating these daily practices into your life, you can cultivate a holistic approach to wellness that encompasses physical, mental, and emotional health. This balanced lifestyle fosters resilience, empowering you to face life's challenges with grace and vitality. By adopting these habits, you can support your health holistically, ensuring that you thrive in both mind and body.

Conclusion: Living in Harmony with Nature through Herbal Wisdom

As we conclude this exploration of herbal practices and their profound impact on health and wellness, it is important to reflect on the guiding principle that living in harmony with nature is at the heart of holistic wellness. Herbal wisdom, rooted in centuries of tradition and empirical knowledge, provides us with valuable insights into how we can enhance our lives through natural means.

This book emphasizes the importance of reconnecting with nature, understanding our bodies, and harnessing the power of plants to promote health, vitality, and balance in our daily lives.

Embracing Dr. Barbara O'Neill's holistic philosophy encourages individuals to view health not merely as the absence of disease, but as a vibrant state of well-being that encompasses physical, mental, and emotional dimensions. Dr. O'Neill's teachings remind us that the body has an innate ability to heal itself when supported by proper nutrition, lifestyle choices, and natural remedies.

By incorporating herbal practices into our daily routines, we can foster a deeper connection with our bodies and the natural world around us. The herbs discussed in this book serve as powerful allies, guiding us toward optimal health and offering a path to self-care that respects the needs of our bodies.

Creating a personal practice for lifelong wellness involves intentionality and mindfulness in our approach to health. This practice should be tailored to individual needs and preferences, considering factors such as age, lifestyle, and health goals.

Incorporating herbs, dietary choices, and holistic practices into our daily lives can improve our overall well-being. Whether it's brewing a soothing herbal tea, engaging in regular physical activity, or practicing mindfulness, these small but meaningful actions add up over time and contribute to a resilient and vibrant life.

In addition, as we navigate the complexities of modern life, it is important to remember the importance of self-care and community. Sharing knowledge about herbal remedies, engaging in family wellness practices, and supporting one another on our health journeys can cultivate a nurturing environment.

By fostering connections with others who share similar goals, we create a supportive network that strengthens our commitment to health and wellness.

Living in harmony with nature through herbal wisdom is an empowering journey. It invites us to listen to our bodies, understand the healing properties of plants, and embrace a holistic approach to wellness.

As we integrate these practices into our daily lives, we can experience a profound transformation that resonates with the rhythms of nature and promotes a healthier, more balanced existence.

As you close this book and begin your journey to greater health and well-being, remember that the path to wellness is not a destination, but a lifelong commitment to nurturing your body, mind, and spirit. Embrace the wisdom of nature and let it guide you toward a life of vitality, balance, and harmony.

Your quest for wellness begins with the choices you make every day, and by prioritizing your health and well-being, you can cultivate a vibrant life that thrives in connection with the world around you.

REFERENCES

1. Pursell, JJ. *The Herbal Apothecary: 100 Medicinal Herbs and How to Use Them*. Timber Press, 2015.

2. Green, James. *The Herbal Medicine-Maker's Handbook: A Home Manual*. Crossing Press, 2000.

3. Cech, Richo. *Making Plant Medicine*. Horizon Herbs, 2000.

4. McIntyre, Anne. *The Complete Herbal Tutor: The Definitive Guide to the Principles and Practices of Herbal Medicine*. Gaia Books, 2010.

5. Gladstar, Rosemary. *Rosemary Gladstar's Medicinal Herbs: A Beginner's Guide*. Storey Publishing, 2012.

6. Kloss, Jethro. *Back to Eden: The Classic Guide to Herbal Medicine, Natural Foods, and Home Remedies Since 1939*. Lotus Press, 1939.

7. Levy, Juliette de Bairacli. *Common Herbs for Natural Health*. Ash Tree Publishing, 1974.

8. Fischer-Rizzi, Susanne. *Complete Earth Medicine Handbook: Natural Healing with Herbs, Essential Oils, and Flower Essences*. Sterling Publishing, 1996.

9. Hernandez, Mimi Prunella. *Herbal: 100 Herbs from the World's Healing Traditions*. Ivy Press, 2021.

10. Tierra, Michael. *The Way of Herbs*. Pocket Books, 1998.

11. De la Forêt, Rosalee. *Alchemy of Herbs: Transform Everyday Ingredients into Foods and Remedies that Heal*. Hay House Inc., 2017.

12. Gladstar, Rosemary. *Herbal Recipes for Vibrant Health*. Storey Publishing, 2008.

13. Books, seminars, and lectures by Barbara O'Neill, a renowned natural health educator and naturopath.

INDEX

D

E

F

G

T

V

W

Y

Bonus Page: Video Short Tutorials by Barbara O'Neill

Thank you for joining us on this journey through the world of herbal healing and natural medicine. To enrich your learning experience, we're thrilled to offer you exclusive access to a collection of video short tutorials featuring Barbara O'Neil. These tutorials, extracted directly from her lectures, provide practical, visual guidance on implementing the natural health practices discussed in this book.

By subscribing, you'll not only gain instant access to our current video library but also be updated with new videos as we continue to add to our collection. This is a fantastic way to stay connected with the latest in herbal healing and natural medicine, ensuring you're always equipped with the knowledge to support your wellness journey.

How to Access:

Simply scan the QR code below or follow the provided link to subscribe and unlock your access. This is our way of saying thank you and enhancing your journey toward holistic health with the invaluable wisdom of Barbara O'Neill.

@INFINITEWELLNESSWAVE

https://www.instagram.com/infinitewellnesswave

As new tutorials become available, you'll be the first to know, allowing you to continuously expand your understanding and application of natural health principles.

We hope these video tutorials serve as a valuable resource in your quest for wellness, bringing the teachings of Barbara O'Neill to life in a new and engaging way. Your feedback and suggestions are always welcome as we grow this library together.

A Message From The Publisher

Are you enjoying the book?
We would love to hear your thoughts!

Many readers do not know how hard reviews are to come by and how much they help a publisher. We would be incredibly grateful if you could take just a few seconds to write a brief review on Amazon, even if it's just a few sentences!

Please go here to leave a quick review:
https://amazon.com/ryp

We would greatly appreciate it if you could take the time to post your review of the book and share your thoughts with the community. If you have enjoyed the book, please let us know what you loved the most about it and if you would recommend it to others. Your feedback is valuable to us, and it helps us to improve our services and continue to offer high-quality literature to our readers.

www.abetteryoueveryday.com

Made in the USA
Middletown, DE
22 December 2024